aquapress

# THE SPORTS DIVING MEDICAL

The definitive guide
to medical conditions
relevant to diving

CHARLES PAUL AZZOPARDI & JOHN PARKER

THIRD REVISED EDITION

An AquaPress Book
Published by AquaPress Ltd
25 Farriers Way
Temple Farm Industrial Estate
Southend-on-Sea
Essex SS2 5RY
United Kingdom

First Published 2023
AquaPress and the AquaPress Logo are Trademarks of AquaPress Ltd.

A CIP catalogue record for this book is available from the British Library.

Diving is an inherently dangerous sport. The information contained in this book is supplied merely for the convenience of the reader and should not be used as the sole source of information. This book is not a substitute for proper training by a recognized diver training agency. The author and publisher have made every effort to ensure that the information in this book is correct at the time of going to press. However, they accept no liability or responsibility whatsoever for any loss, damage, accident, injury or inconvenience sustained by any person using this book or following advice presented in it, provided that this shall not limit or exclude liability for death or personal injury caused by their negligence.

For information on all other AquaPress titles visit www.aquapress.co.uk



ISBN: 978-1-905492473

# FOREWORD

There are few issues in diving medicine as potentially difficult as decision-making around the medical suitability of diving candidates (or sometimes divers themselves) to dive. The aspirations of highly motivated candidates often collide with concerns about medical conditions they may suffer, and these 'concerns' are all too often poorly informed by evidence. In this evidence vacuum, the traditional prescriptive approach to decision-making in 'fitness to dive' consultations often resulted in conservative, risk-averse decisions that would deny diving to candidates whose risk implied by their medical condition was almost certainly small. An unfortunate consequence of this approach was to encourage doctor shopping and withholding of health information by candidates.

Evolution in this space has seen the emergence of a 'discretionary' paradigm in which the diving-related risks implied by a medical condition are analysed as comprehensively as existing evidence allows, and then clearly explained to the candidate. If those risks are not deemed excessive for either the candidate or the people he or she may dive with, then the candidate is endorsed to proceed with diving as an informed risk acceptor. The principal difficulty with this approach is that the assessing doctor requires reasonably detailed knowledge not only of medicine but also of diving and its potential problems.

Even with such knowledge, the evaluation of how a medical condition and diving might interact can be difficult. In the previous two editions of 'The Sports Diving Medical,' Dr John Parker provided the diving community with a tool that substantially reduced that difficulty. After providing some background on diving and its physical and physiological challenges, these works analysed the risk implied in diving by a wide range of medical circumstances and conditions. Risks were stratified according to the level of certainty that the risk exists, the likelihood of the risk occurring, and the severity of consequences if the risk did occur. This formed an extremely strong basis for related discussions with divers and a fantastic aide memoir for even the most experienced diving physicians.

In this third edition, coming more than 20 years after the second, Dr Parker has joined forces with Dr Charles Paul Azzopardi, a research-active, experienced diving physician who practices in Malta, a hub of intense diving activity. Together they have modernized, updated and expanded the text while retaining the key features that made the earlier editions so exquisitely useful. Over the years I have used the previous editions countless times to help channel my thinking on difficult cases. I predict that an entirely new generation of diving physicians will come to see this new edition as indispensable.

Prof Simon Mitchell

## DR CHARLES PAUL AZZOPARDI

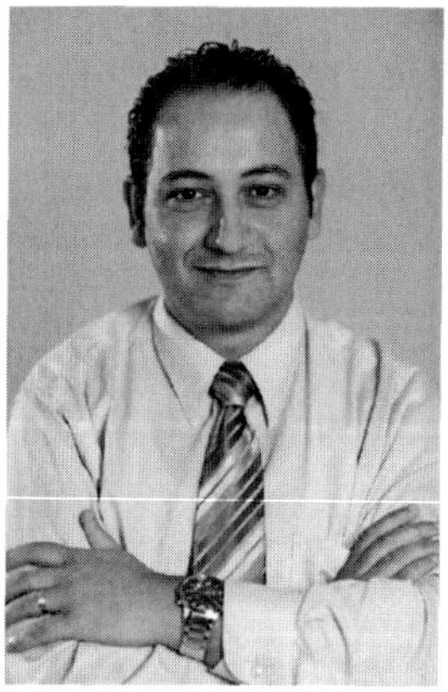

Dr Azzopardi studied medicine in Malta before starting his training in diving and hyperbaric medicine in Plymouth at the Diving Diseases Research Centre (DDRC) in 2016. He then returned to Malta to work at the Mater Dei Hospital Hyperbaric Unit, with rotations in Critical Care / ITU, Anaesthesia, Cardiology and ENT, graduating with a Certificate of Completion of Specialist Training in Baromedicine. He holds postgraduate degrees in Underwater Medicine and Hyperbaric Medicine from the University of Stellenbosch, South Africa. He is an avid sidemount diver and an internationally-awarded photographer in his free time, having published 45 photography coffee table books and the Immediate Past President of the Malta Institute of Professional Photography.

## DR JOHN PARKER

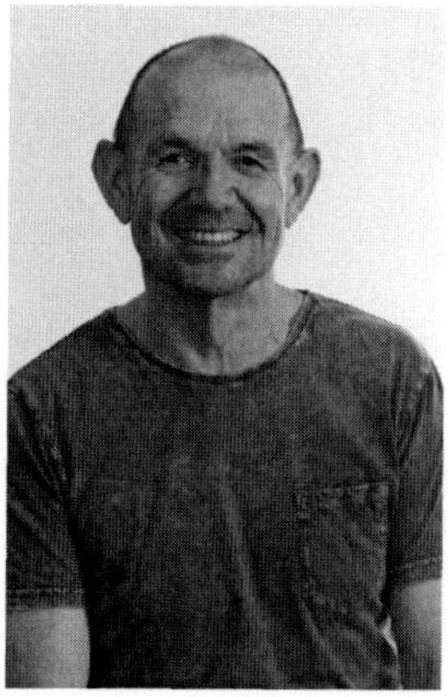

Dr John Parker was born and bred in Liverpool, UK and medically trained at Edinburgh University. He came to Australia to scuba dive the Great Barrier Reef and never returned. He commenced a medical practice in Airlie Beach in Queensland to follow a passion for diving medicine and later worked at Golden Beach in Caloundra on the Sunshine Coast. Intermittently he has ventured with the Red Cross and MSF on humanitarian medical missions including 3 war zones, 2 epidemics and several refugee camps. He spent a year as an expedition medical officer at Davis Station in Antarctica. He is presently working medical locums on Thursday Island in the Torres Straits. He has written earlier editions of 'The Sports Diving Medical", "Poetic Prescriptions for Feeling Good" (2004) and "From Cholera to Ebola: confessions of a humanitarian doctor" (2020).

# PREFACE TO THE 3RD EDITION

'The times, they are a-changing'. Bob Dylan was way ahead of his time as change is ever-accelerating .... hence this new edition of 'The Sports Diving Medical'.

The sport of diving has changed. No longer is it a fringe, extreme activity. It has become a mainstream adventure experience, competing alongside sky diving, mountain biking, snowboarding, canyoning, bungee jumping, abseiling, hand gliding and kiteboarding amongst many others.

It may have lost some of its popularity but divers have increased in diversity, and there is an expanded distribution of older and younger divers. Fifty years ago, there were few 'old divers'. Many of the divers of the sixties and seventies are still diving (us included) and have acquired medical conditions that may affect our diving fitness. Divers as young as eight years of age now commonly venture underwater. More and more divers are learning to dive or experiencing a 'resort dive' on overseas holidays in warm and tropical waters, where prices are cheaper and health and safety are less vigorous.

More divers are using gases other than air. Nitrox is now a common breathing gas once cloistered under the umbrella of 'technical diving'. Technical diving has expanded into the world of closed-circuit rebreathers, with Trimix and Heliox allowing divers to venture deeper and longer. Cave diving too has expanded its reach, popularity and complexity.

Diving for the disabled has become commonplace. Specific professional organizations have been formed to provide specific training courses for divers, instructors and assistants. 'Swapping wheelchair for water' is now an outdated catch cry, as quadriplegics and intellectually disabled persons are given a more accessible underwater experience.

Diving equipment has improved. There is a wider range of sizes and styles. Regulators are more reliable and less 'demanding'. Masks are low volume and better fitting. Full-face masks, once the prerogative of the commercial diver, have dropped in cost and allow better protection of the airway and easy verbal communication between divers and the dive boat. Buoyancy compensators are better fitted and streamlined. Diving computers are smaller, more accurate and user-friendly, although they should never be a substitute for the computer between one's ears, especially knowing that not even the most advanced diving computer has a direct connection with your tissue inert gas levels.

The internet and social media have completely transformed communication, connection and commerce. The smartphone has provided a mobile, instant and affordable platform for immediate access to information, opinion and service. Divers are readily able to access articles, forums and blogs on medical conditions and their relevance to diving. Divers no longer accept a prescriptive decision by a diving specialist physician and will demand an evidence-based justification, which may be particularly hard to come by in the diving medicine setting. Many restrictions for diving are based on expert opinion in the absence of hard data.

Old myths about diving safety are being challenged and busted. Asthma is no longer a blanket contraindication. Diabetics have created protocols to allow them to dive safely. Divers with treated coronary artery disease are returning to diving. The jury is still out on returning to diving after pulmonary and inner ear barotrauma.

Medicine has changed. General practice is no longer 'general' and encompasses more and more niches of expertise – from sports medicine to travel medicine and obviously, diving medicine. The medical and surgical investigation, diagnosis and treatment have evolved dramatically with improved imaging, biomechanical prostheses, endoscopic and robotic surgery, and myriad new medications and immunomodulatory therapies, to mention just a few.

Some things have not changed. Diving-related fatalities continue unabated. The most common causative factors remain non-medical, with separation from buddies and diving beyond one's diving training level being common factors (Lippman). Failure to drop a weight belt and buoyancy problems reflect ongoing deficiencies in training regimes. Poorly maintained equipment is a frequent factor. Stupidity keeps rearing its ugly head – "nothing is foolproof to a talented fool". But medical conditions, particularly cardiac conditions, immersion pulmonary oedema and obesity, do still cause and contribute to many diving incidents and deaths. There is still an important demand for divers to be aware of how their health and fitness level can be critical in the unforgiving and unbreathable hostile underwater environment.

A diving medical assessment is no longer just a simple decision by a doctor as to whether someone is 'fit or unfit to dive'. Instead, it needs to be a risk assessment process, involving the physical and mental health of the diver, the type of diving proposed, the environment in which the dive will occur and the other stakeholders involved in the dive. Once risks have been identified and quantified, there can be an informed discussion as to how they may be mitigated and what conditions and limitations are indicated. The risks can then be accepted or declined by the stakeholders.

So yes ... 'the times, they are changing' and I consider it opportune to review, update and refresh "The Sports Diving Medical". I have humbly seen the wisdom and sought help with this edition. I am grateful to Charles Paul Azzopardi for joining me wholeheartedly in this endeavour. We decided to maintain the original outline of the book after receiving positive feedback about its user-friendly format. Hopefully, with two heads instead of one there will be a wider outlook and output.

The medical sections are organised to follow this thought process.

Each specific risk for a condition of which we are aware is highlighted.

How we might describe the risk is in italics and bracketed, e.g. (a possible, rare and major risk). Many risks are too broad to usefully describe. In those cases, we have not included any comments. How the risk may be reduced is detailed.

Finally, we have put our thoughts and approaches about the condition and what we might do. We include this only as a guide. It is up to everyone to make up their mind.

## FURTHER READING:

Lippmann J, Stevenson C, Taylor D McD. Scuba diving fatalities in Australia, 2001 to 2013: Diver demographics and characteristics. Diving and Hyperbaric Medicine. 2020 June 30;50(2):105–114. doi: 10.28920/dhm50.2.105-114. PMID: 32557411.

**DISCLAIMER**

Recommendations have been made by the authors regarding the fitness to dive. These are only the authors' opinions and should not be taken as gospel. If there is any doubt about a person's fitness to dive, the doctor should refer the case to a qualified and experienced specialist in diving medicine.

In addition, since diving medicine is a relatively new and fast-developing field, the reader is strongly advised to read new literature as it is released and, if necessary, to reassess areas of this book accordingly.

# Contents

# 1

# Risk Assessment & Acceptance

**Diving is an adventure sport. By nature, there are inherent risks to health and life. Anybody who goes diving must therefore accept a risk, whether they are healthy or not. It is the function of the diving medicine specialist to assist the potential diver in assessing the risk, deciding whether it is acceptable and, if it is acceptable, how they can minimise the risk.**

Risk acceptance depends on several factors:

### 1. The risk itself

- The reality of the risk
- The severity of the risk
- The frequency of the risk

### 2. The perception of the risk, which is dependent on

- The level of knowledge of the diver (often of both diving medicine and diving)
- The level of knowledge of the doctor (often of diving and sometimes of diving medicine)

### 3. The level of risk acceptable

- To the diver
- To the doctor
- To the diving instructor or dive school

With so many variables it is no wonder that medical opinion of "fitness to dive" is so subjective, diverse and divisive. For medical opinion to become more consistent and reliable, it is useful to try and describe the risk rather than quantify it with no reliable data.

## THE RISK ITSELF

### a) The reality of the risk

There is little data on the risks of various medical conditions for diving. A risk may be classified as:

**POSSIBLE:** There is a theoretical concern that the medical condition could cause a significant problem to health or life whilst diving but there is little anecdotal or scientific evidence to support it.

After radial keratotomy of the cornea, there is a "possible" (theoretical) risk of rupture of the eyeball from a mask squeeze but there has never been a recorded case.

**PLAUSIBLE:** There is very strong theoretical or anecdotal evidence that this condition could cause a risk to health or life.

If a diver has pleural adhesions there is a "plausible" increased risk of cerebral arterial gas embolism. There are case reports to support it but no reliable scientific data.

**PROVEN:** There is good scientific evidence or overwhelming anecdotal evidence to prove that the medical condition is a risk to health or life.

There is strong scientific evidence to support the claim that the incidence of middle ear barotrauma while diving with an upper respiratory infection is increased, which is "proven".

### b) The frequency of a risk occurring

If a risk is valid then what is the likelihood of it happening?

**REGULAR:** The risk has a high chance of occurring if you take it.

**REMOTE:** The risk has a small chance of occurring if you take it.

**RARE:** The risk rarely occurs if you take it.

If a diver goes scuba diving with a sinus infection there is a "regular" risk of sinus barotrauma, a "remote" risk of orbital haematoma and a "rare" risk of a pneumocephalus.

### c) The severity of the risk

Should the risk be accepted as valid, then the severity of the risk needs to be assessed. Is the risk:

**MILD:** If the risk happens, then only minor bodily injury will occur and should heal with little danger of long-term injury.

Diving with a cold may cause a "mild" middle ear barotrauma which causes pain and reduced hearing for a week or two but which normally heals with full resolution.

**MODERATE:** If the risk eventuates then moderate injury will occur that may leave a permanent disability.

Diving with a cold may cause a "moderate" inner ear barotrauma with a round window fistula which could leave permanent hearing loss.

**MAJOR:** If the risk eventuates there will be a serious injury, with a risk of severe long-term disability or loss of life.

Diving with a past medical history of spontaneous pneumothorax may cause a "major" pneumothorax, which could easily lead to loss of life.

Using these three criteria it is possible to describe a risk (we call it the P/R/M classification).

Reality – Possible / Plausible / Proven
Frequency – Regular / Remote / Rare
Severity – Mild / Moderate / Major

For example, if a diver has a past medical history of recurrent ear infections and there is rigid scarring of the eardrum, the risk of perforation of the ear drum could be described as a plausible, regular and moderate risk.

If a diver has mild angina, the risk of anginal pain with disablement in the water could be described as a proven, regular and major risk.

If a diver has a past medical history of a traumatic pneumothorax from a fractured rib, the risk of recurrent pneumothorax whilst diving could be described as a possible, rare and major risk.

Although there may still be some disagreement upon the classification, it encourages a real breakdown of the risks and there will be a far greater alignment of opinion than just a "fit to dive" or "not fit to dive" assessment.

## THE PERCEPTION OF THE RISK

### a) The level of knowledge of the potential diver

A novice diver may be completely unaware of the dangers of the underwater environment or the effects of increased pressures on the body. They are often quite incredulous when told of possible risks.

When a paraplegic diver was told of the plausible, remote but major risk of increased incidence of decompression illness they were very willing to limit the depth of diving to less than 10 metres.

### b) The level of knowledge of the doctor

The doctor may also be unaware of the dangers of the underwater environment and unless they have extra training in underwater medicine will not appreciate the physics or physiology of increased pressure on the body. It is therefore essential that any doctor doing a diving medical (as with aviation medicine) have recognised postgraduate training and qualifications in diving & hyperbaric medicine.

A diver with exercise-induced asthma was given a medical certificate stating they were fit to dive but should not dive deeper than 10 metres.

## THE LEVEL OF RISK ACCEPTABLE

### a) To the diver

The level of risk acceptable to an individual is variable. An 18-year-old biker will often accept any level of risk, thinking they are immortal. A 35-year-old single mother of three small children will often not undertake any activity with any moderate or major risk, no matter how remote or rare. A 65-year-old widower on a world backpacking trip will accept more risk than the still-married, just-retired pensioner.

### b) To the doctor

Doctors too are quite variable in their acceptance of risk-taking, which transfers to the level of risk they feel their patients should accept. Some doctors are rather paternalistic and consider novice divers to be incapable of understanding the risks and therefore should not take any.

Other doctors may tend to be avant-garde and be readily influenced by "soft statistics" and encourage divers to take a risk over natural caution. Doctors with little experience in diving medicine, fearful of litigation, may be very conservative in endorsing risk-taking. Certainly, in the second millennium far more of the medical profession will allow their patients to take an informed risk.

## c) To the diving school or company

A diver may arrive for a course with a medical certificate of "fitness to dive" but with which they do not agree. Alternatively, when filling out the predive forms and medical questionnaire, a medical condition may be noted, which the diving instructor knows to be a major risk factor. As the diving instructor has a duty of care to the diver, the other divers on the course or trip and the diving company, they have to decide whether they too accept the risk or seek further medical opinion.

An important part of any diving medical is therefore the explanation of the risk and a discussion of its acceptance. Rather than classify a diver as "fit to dive" or "not fit to dive" it is preferable to state that the medical risks of diving have been described and explained and that the diver understands the possible adverse consequences, accepts those risks and has been informed how to reduce those risks.

The doctor has a duty of care to prevent a diver from taking foolhardy risks and there will be some disagreement between doctors and divers on these boundaries. However, we believe using such a method of describing a risk will encourage a more thorough, consistent and uniform process of risk assessment. In our view, this can only enhance the consistency of outcomes.

Most divers will heed the advice of the doctor and follow recommendations. The doctor should document the advice given.

## We have 6 levels of comfort into which we find our medical recommendations may broadly fall.

1. This person has a very significant risk. It is dangerous for them to dive at any time and there is no way we would agree to them diving whatever risk they are willing to accept, e.g., an uncontrolled epileptic.
2. This person has a very significant risk, which could be dangerous. The risk will lessen in time and we would not agree with them diving until the risk has fallen to a more acceptable level, e.g., a recent head injury.
3. This person is chronically unable to look after themselves or others underwater. There is no way we would freely recommend diving. The increased risks could be reduced in a fully supervised, carefully controlled and exceedingly conservative diving environment. If the person understands and accepts the risks and agrees to stay within that defined diving environment, we would then agree to them diving, e.g., a paraplegic or blind person.
4. This person has a significant, currently stable risk but potentially could become quickly unstable. There is no way we would freely agree to diving. The present risk could be reduced following protocols designed for the condition. If the person understands and accepts the risks, agrees to stay within that defined diving environment and agrees to stop diving should their risk become unstable, we would then agree to them diving, e.g. a well-controlled insulin-dependent diabetic.
5. This person is able-bodied and has a theoretical risk which is probably not a real risk but we cannot guarantee it is not real. No data exists. The diver should know about it just in case it does occur. If they accept that risk, we would agree to them diving, e.g., hypertension.
6. This person has no obvious significant risk from their medical status and we agree to them diving, e.g., after a radial keratotomy.

## THE SPORT

**Diving is a unique sport. It is vastly different from any other adventure sport. The underwater environment moves in all directions with the tide, current and wave action. These movements can change dramatically and unpredictably, even during a dive. What starts as a gentle swim can end in an exhausting finning marathon. Getting in the water may be easy but getting out may become difficult and dangerous from swell or wave action that may suddenly occur from a change in tide. The diver cannot always have a rest when tired.**

The underwater environment is unbreathable. At all times underwater the diver is dependent on a self-contained breathing apparatus with an adequate supply of respirable gas, e.g., air or mixed gases. The underwater environment exposes the body to numerous and sometimes novel stresses:

### COLD

- The body cools more quickly in water than in air.
- Every diver will get cold, especially towards the end of the dive.
- When the face is immersed in cold water, there is a reflex slowing of the heart rate, apnoea and vasoconstriction (the diving reflex)

### ANXIETY

- Especially in novice divers who are unsure of what to expect.
- The unpredictable often happens during a dive, so even the experienced diver can become anxious.
- There are many dangers underwater, some real and many expectant.

### SENSORY DEPRIVATION

**Reduced vision:**

- The mask restricts peripheral vision.
- Dirty water limits visibility.
- The visual horizons can be lost when in very clear or very dirty water.
- Colours are lost with depth.
- It gets darker with depth.

**Reduced hearing:**

- Localisation of sound is lost.
- A diving hood may occlude the ear.
- Reduced touch; cold hands or gloves diminish feeling.

## REDUCED BALANCE

Weightlessness can disturb balance.

## UPSIDE-DOWN POSITIONS

When weightless, the body can be easily placed in unusual positions whilst the body contents, especially in the abdomen, are still subject to the forces of gravity.

## PRESSURE

All the air spaces in the body must continually equalise to the constantly changing ambient pressure. Failure to do so will quickly result in tissue damage (barotrauma).

Breathing air at high pressure can have harmful effects from each of its components:

Nitrogen can become narcotic when diving deeper than about 30 m (100 ft), causing a reduction in judgement and concentration. Decompression illness is caused by the formation of nitrogen bubbles in tissues when the diver exceeds depth/time limits and ascends too quickly. Carbon dioxide can become toxic if a build-up occurs through skip breathing, mechanical resistance of equipment, increased density of air and exertion. This might aggravate nitrogen narcosis and precipitate oxygen toxicity.

Oxygen can also become acutely toxic, causing convulsions if breathed at high pressures. Fortunately, this does not occur when breathing air in less than 50 m (165 ft) but it becomes relevant when diving deeper on air or breathing gas mixtures with higher concentrations of oxygen, e.g., nitrox or enriched air diving.

No other sport gives such a variety of stresses, so frequently, in such complex combinations and over such short periods.

# THE PHYSICS

The basic physics of diving are always worthy of revision.

## THE PRESSURE EXERTED ON A DIVER

The air (or atmospheric) pressure at sea level is one atmosphere (atm) of pressure. The water pressure exerted by 10 metres (33 feet) of seawater also equals one atmosphere. The total (or absolute) pressure exerted on a diver is the sum of the air and water pressures. It is termed atmosphere absolute.

| Depth in metres | Depth in feet | Air pressure | Water pressure | Atmospheres Absolute |
|---|---|---|---|---|
| Surface | Surface | 1 atm | nil | 1 ATA |
| 10 | 33 | 1 atm | 1 atm | 2 ATA |
| 20 | 66 | 1 atm | 2 atm | 3 ATA |
| 30 | 99 | 1 atm | 3 atm | 4 ATA |
| 40 | 132 | 1 atm | 4 atm | 5 ATA |
| 90 | 297 | 1 atm | 9 atm | 10 ATA |

The pressure exerted on a diver is easily calculated from the formula:

Pressure = (depth in metres /10) + 1 (in ATA)

## PASCAL'S PRINCIPLE

The solid and liquid parts of the diver's body are considered incompressible over the range of pressures encountered during sports diving. Any pressure is therefore transmitted through them with no distortion or damage. Hence the water pressure pushes onto the skin, which pushes on to fat, which pushes on to muscle with no distortion or damage to those tissues. This does not apply to the gas spaces in the body, the ears, sinuses, lungs, and intestines, which all contain air and are compressible. Any increased external pressure will squeeze these spaces unless the air pressure within them is also increased equally.

## BOYLE'S LAW

The volume of a gas is inversely proportional to its absolute pressure at a constant temperature.

This is the gas law most relevant to diving. As the diver descends and the pressure increases, the volume of any gas space in the body decreases proportionally. What most new divers do not realise is that the greatest rate of change of volume occurs in the first few metres of a dive. This is best demonstrated by plotting the absolute pressure against volume.

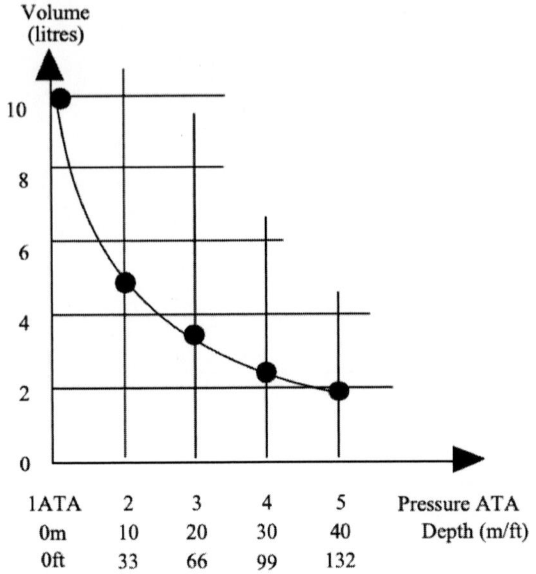


Whenever the pressure within an air-containing cavity of the body differs from the surrounding pressure, the volume of that cavity will be squeezed or stretched in accordance with Boyle's Law. If the squeezing or stretching goes beyond the normal elasticity of that tissue then trauma will occur. This damage is called barotrauma.

There are two types of barotrauma:

Barotrauma of descent – this occurs when, on the descent, the ambient pressure becomes greater than the pressure within the air-containing cavity. This commonly occurs in the middle ear cavity, when the tympanic membrane becomes inwardly stretched until it will eventually perforate, with water entering the middle ear cavity to reduce the volume and equalise the pressure. At the same time, the mucosal lining of the middle cavity becomes oedematous and haemorrhages so that blood accumulates in the cavity, reducing its volume and thereby equalising the pressure.

Barotrauma of ascent – this occurs when, on the ascent, the pressure within the air-containing cavity becomes greater than the external pressure and cannot readily and passively escape. In the lung, such an air expansion can cause hyperinflation of the lung tissue to the point of maximum elasticity, when it will tear at its weakest point. The expanding air will follow the path of least tissue resistance and cause mediastinal emphysema and/or pneumothorax and/or enter the bloodstream causing an arterial gas embolism (AGE). So-called pulmonary barotrauma of ascent can occur with as little transpulmonary overpressure of 75 cm (30 inches) of water and has occurred in swimming pools. Because the greatest rate of change of volume is near the surface, most barotraumatic injuries occur near the surface. Depth restriction will therefore not reduce the risk of barotrauma during a dive.

## DALTON'S LAW

The total pressure exerted by a mixture of gases is the sum of the pressures that would be exerted by each of the gases if it alone occupied the total volume.

Using this law, it is possible to calculate the partial pressure (pp) of each component of air at any depth. Assuming the composition of air to be simplified as 20% oxygen and 80% nitrogen:

| Depth in metres | Depth in feet | Absolute Pressure ATA | Pp of Nitrogen ATA | Pp of Oxygen ATA |
|---|---|---|---|---|
| Surface | Surface | 1 | 0.8 | 0.2 |
| 10 | 33 | 2 | 1.6 | 0.4 |
| 20 | 66 | 3 | 2.4 | 0.6 |
| 30 | 99 | 4 | 3.2 | 0.8 |
| 40 | 132 | 5 | 4.0 | 1.0 |
| 70 | 231 | 8 | 6.4 | 1.6 |

This law explains the toxic effects of gases at depth.

### Nitrogen narcosis

Nitrogen is inert at normal pressures but as its partial pressure increases it becomes narcotic. This is commonly encountered when diving at depths greater than 30 m (100 ft) and the narcosis becomes more pronounced as the pressure increases. The effects include impairment of judgement, concentration and memory, a sense of well-being, light-headedness and anxiety. It can eventually lead to unconsciousness. The overall effect is similar to drunkenness. It is the most significant factor limiting the depth of safe recreational air diving.

### Oxygen toxicity

Oxygen too will become toxic if breathed for extended periods at higher-than-normal pressures. Partial pressures of oxygen as low as 1.2 ATA can produce convulsions although an oxygen partial pressure of 1.5 ATA (equivalent to a depth of about 60 m (200 ft) when breathing air) is regarded as generally safe.

## HENRY'S LAW

The amount of gas that will dissolve in a liquid is directly proportional to the partial pressure of that gas over the liquid at any given temperature.

Using this law, it is possible to begin to calculate the amount of nitrogen taken up by the body during diving. It is most relevant in explaining decompression illness. The longer and the deeper the dive, the greater the amount of nitrogen that is absorbed into the tissues of the body. If decompression is too rapid, this extra nitrogen will come out of the solution before it can be exhaled from the lungs, causing a plethora of symptoms. The more common symptoms of decompression illness are weakness, pain in the joints and muscles, mental dullness, paraesthesia, numbness, headache, a skin rash, dizziness and nausea.

# THE DIVERS

Divers can be divided into seven broad groups:

## RESORT DIVER

One who dives on a single day, under strict professional supervision, in optimal water conditions, according to an extremely conservative dive plan.

## RECREATIONAL or SPORTS DIVER

One who dives solely on compressed air for pleasure and who can choose the time, place and plan of the dive.

## TECHNICAL DIVER

One who dives solely for pleasure but who extends the limits of recreational diving to new frontiers, e.g., deep penetration cave divers, diving using various gas mixtures and more complex equipment, e.g., closed circuit rebreathers.

## PROFESSIONAL INSTRUCTIONAL DIVER

One who dives for employment in instruction and/or supervision of divers, e.g., divemasters, diving supervisors, and diving instructors.

## PROFESSIONAL OCCUPATIONAL DIVERS

One who dives for employment, the nature of which determines the time, place and plan of their dive, e.g., scientific divers, fish farm divers, abalone divers, and police divers.

## COMMERCIAL DIVERS (not implying that they are not professional or occupational)

One who dives for employment using various gases and equipment, often involving hard manual work and in exacting conditions, e.g., harbour divers, and oil rig divers.

## MILITARY DIVERS

One who dives under the jurisdiction of the armed forces, highly disciplined and trained with a variety of specialised equipment for the toughest of conditions.

The mental and physical demands and the responsibilities of each of these groups differ dramatically and the medical standards for each must reflect those differences.

**This book is about the recreational sports diver but is also relevant to the resort and technical divers, although diving instructors are truly commercial divers themselves.**

## WHY HAVE A DIVING MEDICAL?

**Diving involves risk, with many being increased by pre-existing medical conditions. Most divers, especially novice divers, have no appreciation of these risks. The main purpose of the diving medical is therefore:**

- to identify any relevant pre-existing medical condition
- to determine the risks that any pre-existing medical condition causes whilst diving and how those risks may be reduced
- to decide whether the risks are acceptable

However, mandatory pre-dive training diving medicals have been abandoned since about 2013 and diving medicals are now only required based on responses to a self-reported medical questionnaire, e.g.

1) RSTC Medical Statement - (see link in the bibliography) - used by BSAC, SAA, SSAC

2) UKDMC Recreational Diving Medical Declaration - (see link in the bibliography) - used by BSAC, SAA, SSAC

Even after an initial diving medical, there is no compulsion for repeat diving medicals as the diver ages. Some diving organisations do insist on annual medical questionnaires and recommend a diving medical at the age of 45 years and every five years thereafter until the age of 65 years when an annual diving medical is recommended.

Diving medicals are also often recommended after any major medical event.

Many divers now only dive on commercial diving trips and often buddy up with a total stranger. Any diver needs to be confident that their buddy is medically fit and appropriately trained so they do not add risk to themselves. It is also preferable that the buddy is of similar fitness, experience and interest so no diver is forced to dive beyond their capabilities.

## THE SPORTS DIVING MEDICAL

This should consist of:

- A questionnaire
- An interview with the diver to discuss the completed questionnaire
- A physical examination
- Investigations
- Discussion on the risks involved, the risks acceptable and ways to reduce the risks.

## 1. THE QUESTIONNAIRE

There are various questionnaires in use around the world, including:

- UKDMC Recreational Diving Medical Declaration (see link in the bibliography)
- Recreational Scuba Training Council (RSTC) Medical Statement - (see link in the bibliography)
- South Pacific Underwater Medicine Society (SPUMS) medical questionnaire (see link in the bibliography)

We use the SPUMS medical questionnaire.

## 2. THE INTERVIEW

This should expand and elucidate the positive answers given in the questionnaire. This book may help select further questions. Certain questions on the questionnaire promote useful discussion, e.g.,

- The use of contact lenses or glasses leads to a discussion on the possible problems encountered with contact lenses underwater and the use of masks with prescriptive lenses.
- A history of ear pain whilst flying leads to a more detailed assessment and explanation of ear equalisation techniques.
- History of back pain leads to a discussion on lifting techniques with heavy diving equipment.

## 3. THE EXAMINATION

This must be thorough and take special note of the air-containing cavities of the body. The following are the authors' routines and are included as a guide only.

Weight, height, calculation of body mass index (BMI), visual acuity.

**GENERAL** – during the examination specifically look for scars, muscle wasting and weakness, agility and mobility whilst dressing and getting on and off the couch.

**MENTAL HEALTH** – despite the brevity of the medical, it is important to assess maturity, psychological stability and psychiatric state. Inappropriate comments, actions or behaviour should be a warning (alas there is no screening test for stupidity).

### Whilst the patient is sitting:

**SKIN** – colour, rashes.

**BLOOD PRESSURE** – if high, repeat with the patient lying down after a short rest. If any concerns remain, a 24-hour ambulatory BP test is usually informative.

**PULSE** – rate, rhythm and volume.

**MOUTH** – ulceration, palate deformities, bifid uvula, gingivitis, movement of the soft palate (IX), tongue movement (X).

**THROAT and TONSILS** – infection, post-nasal discharge.

**TEETH** – caries, conditions of fillings, fitting of dental and orthodontic appliances.

**NASAL PASSAGES** – patency (get the diver to sniff through each nostril), septal deviation, polyps, discharge, mucosal colour.

**EYES** – the presence of contact lenses, ptosis, nystagmus, pupillary reflexes to light and accommodation, and eye movements (III, IV and VI).

**FACE** – rashes, e.g., herpes simplex, facial movements (VII), facial sensation (V).

### With the patient standing:

**EARS** – External ears – hearing aid, wax or debris (wash or suck out if ear canal occluded), infection, exostosis.

**Tympanic membrane** – scarring, perforation, retraction, effusion, barotrauma, monomeric area (which bulges like a balloon when the ear is equalised).

**Eustachian tube** – ask the diver to perform a Valsalva manoeuvre whilst you are watching the light reflex on the tympanic membrane. A movement of the membrane will usually be seen. See Appendix A.

### With the diver is undressed and lying on the couch:

**NECK** – cervical lymphadenopathy, enlarged thyroid, central trachea, increased jugular venous pressure, carotid bruits.

**HEART** – displaced apex beat, thrills, normal heart sounds.

**CHEST** – deformities, scars on the chest wall from surgery or drains, normal respiratory movements, normal chest percussion, normal breath sounds whilst the diver is forcibly hyperventilating through an open mouth (to enhance any rhonchi).

**SPINE** – deformities, scars.

**ABDOMEN** – scars, splenic or hepatic enlargement, masses, hernia, inguinal lymphadenopathy, abdominal bruits

**NERVOUS SYSTEM** – muscle wasting, normal coordination, equal and normal reflexes, normal muscle strength.

**PERIPHERAL VASCULAR SYSTEM** – normal pulses in legs, skin abnormalities on lower legs.

## SHARPENED ROMBERG TEST (SRT)

Many diving doctors include this test in their medical. It is a useful test in the assessment of divers with possible decompression illness. This manoeuvre narrows the proprioceptive base and places a severe strain on the labyrinthine function. The diver stands with their feet aligned in tandem heel-to-toe (preferably in bare feet and on a hard floor), crossing their arms with their hands on the opposite shoulder, closing their eyes and remaining still for up to 60 seconds. The time that the diver remains balanced is noted. The most consistent and sensitive method of measuring the SRT is to record the longest time of four attempts.

**SERIAL SEVENS** – Some doctors record a serial seven score as a baseline for mental agility. It can be an aid in diagnosing decompression illness. The diver must, out loud, subtract seven from one hundred and keep on subtracting seven from the answer. The time taken to complete the test is noted. 100…93…86…79…72…65…58…51…44…37…30…23…16…9…2 If the diver gives an incorrect answer the doctor should quickly correct it.

The number of mistakes and the time taken should be recorded. A diver who completes the exercise in 57 seconds with two mistakes would be recorded as 2 mistakes/57secs. A diver who makes no mistakes and takes 1 min and 20 seconds would be recorded as 0 mistakes/80secs. Having repeated the test several times on numerous divers over many years we are impressed by the consistency of the results.

## 4. NORMAL INVESTIGATIONS

The sensitivity and specificity of most screening investigations in the diving medical are low and there has been much discussion as to their true value. However, the following investigations are still recommended.

**URINALYSIS** – all divers should have their urine tested for protein and glucose to detect any undiagnosed diabetes or renal disease.

**PULMONARY FUNCTION TESTING** – to try and detect any clinical or sub-clinical restrictive or obstructive lung disease all divers should have spirometry to measure their forced vital capacity (FVC), forced expiratory volume in one second ($FEV_1$) and their ratio of $FEV_1$/ FVC. Normal predicted values are calculated for age, height, sex and race. For a guide to lung function see Appendix C.

**AUDIOMETRY** – air audiometry covering the frequencies 0.25 Hz to 8 Hz is recommended if there is a history or sign of hearing loss, middle ear or inner ear pathology. It will also act as a baseline for future assessments. But ongoing routine audiograms are not justified in future medicals unless the diver is symptomatic. (Hausmann)

**CHEST X-RAY** – a chest X-ray is only recommended for any diver with a medical history, symptom or sign of serious or recurrent lung infection, a medical history of disease with possible pulmonary complications, a family history of tuberculosis, an occupational history with a high risk of lung disease, medical history of mechanical ventilation or unexplained abnormal lung function tests.

However, in a study of 15 consecutive cases of pulmonary barotrauma, 5 cases of subpleural emphysematous blebs were noted on CT scans which were not detected in pre-injury or post-injury chest X-rays. When cystic lung disease is suspected a high-definition spiral lung CT scan should be advised (Russi, Reuter).

**TYMPANOGRAM** – is recommended for any diver who cannot demonstrate auto-inflation of the middle ear with repeated attempts. It may help to elucidate whether there is middle ear pathology present.

**PREGNANCY TEST** – is recommended for any female diver who is late with their menstrual period and could be pregnant.

**STANDARD VALIDATED CARDIOVASCULAR RISK ASSESSMENT**, e.g. NVDPA 'Australian Absolute CV disease risk calculator'. All divers 45 years and older, or anyone younger with multiple risk factors, should have this assessment. Anyone with a risk >10% is advised to further have an exercise stress ECG or echocardiogram and/or, if possible, a coronary angiogram.

**ELECTROCARDIOGRAM (ECG)** – is recommended for all asymptomatic divers.

**EXERCISE TESTING** – as a physician assessing fitness to dive, you should consider conducting a Chester Step Test (CST) to estimate maximal oxygen uptake (VO2 max) to measure the diver's cardiopulmonary fitness and aerobic capacity. The CST is a sub-maximal, multistage aerobic capacity test, using a 25 cm or 30 cm step height.

## 5. DISCUSSION

Any medical condition, pre-existing or discovered by the medical, must be discussed in terms of its relevance and risk for diving:

- Will the condition compromise the diver's safety in the water?
- Will diving make the condition worse or is its treatment less effective?
- Will the condition predispose the diver to a diving-related illness or injury?

The diver must understand the possible adverse outcomes of the risk and the likelihood of it occurring. Methods to reduce the risk should be discussed including whether the reduced risk is acceptable to both the diver and the doctor.

Rather than give a traditional certificate stating whether the diver is 'FIT/UNFIT', it is better to give a 'Statement of Health for Recreational Diving', a statement of findings, advice given and recommendations. (see link - SPUMS Diving Medical Risk assessment for Recreational Divers in the bibliography).

### This should include:

- Diver's full name and address

- Diver's date of birth
- Date of medical
- Standard specification of the medical if appropriate
- A statement to summarise the conclusion of the medical
- A statement that the doctor has explained the risks and that the diver has a good understanding of them
- Advice given to the diver to minimise any risk (if appropriate)
- The doctor's name, address and telephone number
- The doctor's signature
- A signed statement that the diver understands and accepts the findings, conclusions and risks
- A signed statement that the conclusions are dependent on the disclosure of a full medical history

It is then up to the diver to decide their actions and the inherent repercussions thereof.

## FURTHER READING:


1. Baines C. Diving Hyperb Med 2013 Dec;43(4):244-6. Perceptions amongst Tasmanian recreational scuba divers of the value of a diving medical. PMID: 24510335
2. Denoble PJ. DAN Annual Diving Report 2019 Edition: A report on 2017 diving fatalities, injuries, and incidents [Internet]. Durham (NC): Divers Alert Network; 2019. Divers Alert Network Annual Diving Reports. PMID: 32991099 Bookshelf ID: NBK562527
3. Elliott D. Why fitness? Who benefits from Diver Medical Examinations? SPUMS J 2000; 30(4): 204-9
4. Fitzgerald B. A review of the Sharpened Romberg's test in diving medicine. SPUMS J 1996; 26(3): 142-6
5. Fowler B, Ackles K N, Porlieu G. Effects of inert gas narcosis on behaviour: a critical review. Undersea Biomed Res 1985; 12: 369-402
6. Glen S, White S, Douglas J. Medical Supervision of sport diving in Scotland: reassessing the need for routine medical examinations. Br J Sports Med 2000; 34: 375-8
7. Glen S. Br J Sports Med 2004 Dec;38(6):754-7. doi: 10.1136/bjsm.2003.008987. Three-year follow-up of a self-certification system for the assessment of fitness to dive in Scotland. PMID: 15562174 PMCID: PMC1724981 DOI: 10.1136/bjsm.2003.008987
8. Gorman D. Health Surveillance in the 21st Century. SPUMS J 2001; 31(1): 39-41
9. Gorman D. Fitness for Diving: a review of the critical issues. SPUMS J 1994; 24(1): 2-4
10. Halstead B. Assume the risk and take the blame. SPUMS J 1997; 27(3): 153-4
11. Hausmann D, Laabling S, Hoth S, Plinkert PK, Klingmann C. Assessment of the peripheral hearing system of sport divers. Undersea Hyperb Med Nov-Dec 2011;38(6):515-26. Assessment of the peripheral hearing system of sport divers
12. Jarchow T, Mast F W. The effect of water immersion on postural and visual orientation. Aviat Space Environ Med 1999; 70(9): 879-86
13. Jepson N, Rienks R, Smart D, Bennett MH, Mitchell SJ, Turner M.Diving Hyperb Med 2020 Sep 30;50(3):273-277. doi: 10.28920/dhm50.3.273-277. South Pacific Underwater Medicine Society guidelines for cardiovascular risk assessment of divers. PMID: 32957130 DOI: 10.28920/dhm50.3.273-277
14. Lawrence C H. A diving fatality due to oxygen toxicity during a "technical" dive. Med J Aust 1996; 165(2): 262-3

15. Lee C T. Sharpening the Sharpened Rombergs. SPUMS J 1998; 28(3): 125-32

16. Lippman J, Stevenson C, McD Taylor D, Williams J. Diving Hyperb Med 2016 Dec;46(4):241-246. Estimating the risk of a scuba diving fatality in Australia. PMID: 27966203

17. Meehan C, Bennett M. Diving Hyperb Med 2010 Sep;40(3):119-24. Medical assessment of fitness to dive - comparing a questionnaire and a medical interview-based approach. PMID: 23111909

18. Reuter M, Tetzlaff K, Warninghoff V, Steffens J C, Bettinghausen E, Heller M. Computed tomography of the chest in diving-related pulmonary barotrauma. Br J Radiol 1997; 70(833): 440-5

19. Richardson D. The RSTC Medical Statement and Candidate Screening Model. SPUMS J 2000; 30(4): 210-3

20. Rienks, R, Buwalda M, Bucx J, Dubois E, Wingelaar T, van Hulst R Cardiovascular risk assessment in divers: Toward safer diving. Undersea Hyperb Med. . 2022 Third Quarter;49(3):355-365. PMID: 36001568

21. Rogers J H. Romberg and his test. J Laryngol Otology 1980; 94: 1401-4

22. RSTC Medical Statement https://www.padi.com/sites/default/files/documents/padi-courses/2.1.5%20rstc%20 medstate%20v201.pdf

23. Russi E W. Diving and the risk of Barotrauma. Thorax 1998; 53 (Suppl 2): S20-4

24. Sames C, Gorman D, Mitchell S, Zhou L. Long-term changes in spirometry in occupational divers: a 10–25 year audit. Diving and Hyperbaric Medicine. 2018 March;48(1):10–16. doi:10.28920/dhm48.1.10-16. PMID: 29557096.

25. Simpson G, Roomes D. Scuba diving medical examinations in practice – a postal survey. Med J Aust 1999; 171(11-12): 595-8

26. SPUMS Diving Medical Risk assessment for Recreational Divers https://spums.org.au/sites/default/files/SPUMS%20 Diving%20Medical%20Forms_2020.pdf

27. St Leger Dowse M, Waterman KM, El Penny C, Smerdon GR. Diving Hyperb Med 2015 Sep;45(3):184-9. Does self-certification reflect the cardiac health of UK sports divers? PMID: 26415070

28. Sykes K. Chester Step Test. Occupational Medicine 2018;68(1):70-71 academic.oup.com/occmed/ article/68/1/70/4866348

29. Taylor D M, O'Toole K S, Auble T E, Ryan C M, Sherman D R. Sensation seeking personality traits of recreational scuba divers. SPUMS J 2001; 31(1): 25-8

30. Taylor DM, Lippmann J, Smith D. The absence of hearing loss in otologically asymptomatic recreational scuba divers. Undersea Hyperb Med. 2006 Mar-Apr;33(2):135-41.

31. Tetzlaff K, Reuter M, Leplow B, Heller M, Bettinghausen E. Risk factors for pulmonary barotrauma in divers. Chest 1997; 112(3): 654-9

32. UKDMC Recreational Diving Medical Declaration http://www.ukdmc.org/wp-content/uploads/2017/04/Medical-Form-Jan-2021-Final-version-31.1.2021-1.pdf

33. Veale A, Richardson D, Gorman D. Draft SPUMS Policy on Medical Practitioner Certification of Fitness for Diving. SPUMS J 1995; 25(4): 214-5

34. Whayne TF. Medical Management and Risk Reduction of the Cardiovascular Effects of Underwater Diving. PMID: 28676021 DOI: 10.2174/1570161115666170621084316

35. Wingelaar TT, Endert EL, Hoencamp R, van Ooij PJAM, van Hulst RA. Longitudinal screening of hearing threshold in navy divers: is diving really a hazard? Diving and Hyperbaric Medicine. 2019 December 20;49(4):283–290. doi: 10.28920/dhm49.4.283-290. PMID: 31828747.

# General issues

# 2

## AGE

**Diving at the extremes of age poses special risks.**

## CHILDREN

- Up to the 1990s scuba diving was recommended only for people aged 16 years plus. Over the years the age has slowly fallen. Now, most training agencies accept children aged 12 or over for open-water training.
- Some instructor agencies give a Junior Open Water Diver Certification at the age of 10 years with a depth restriction of 12 metres.
- Several organisations give children as young as eight years a "diving experience", where they have one-to-one supervision with a diving instructor in clear calm water and depth is restricted to less than 2 meters (Richardson).
- Diving gear (even when designed for children) is bulky and heavy out of the water. Open water diving requires some strength and stamina, especially when kitting up, entering and exiting the water. Some doctors have specified 45 kg (100 lb) and 1.5 m (5 ft) limitations or a requirement to have attained 90% of predicted adult height (Dembert).
- Children have relatively narrower Eustachian tubes and sinus ostia, so may be more susceptible to barotrauma of the middle ear and sinuses. A history of recurrent middle ear infections, ear pain whilst flying, atopy, and previous ENT surgery should be noted.
- Children have a higher incidence of asthma than adults and seem to be more susceptible to broncho-constrictive stimuli e.g., exertion and cold dry air.
- Children have relatively low lung elasticity and airway diameter leading to a higher breathing effort and increased airway collapse at end of expiration compared to adults. In theory, this could make them more vulnerable to pulmonary barotrauma.
- Children have open epiphyses of their long bones. Their growth is accelerated in early adolescence. There is a theoretical concern that the epiphysis could be injured by bubble formation during decompression.
- Children have a high body surface area relative to their metabolic rate, a lower body mass index and relatively less subcutaneous fat than an adult making them more prone to hypothermia. Moreover, the neoprene wetsuit will have a relatively greater effect on buoyancy control for the smaller diver requiring more weights and more buoyancy compensation on descent and ascent.
- Children have a smaller blood volume and lower total body water relative to their body surface area. Sweating will cause dehydration more quickly in children than adults.
- Diving demands good executive functioning, i.e., the cognitive process to control, regulate and manage thoughts and actions. In young adolescents, this is still immature with less ability for sustained attention, cognitive flexibility and concentration (Buwalda).

- Parents can coerce their children to follow the same interests as themselves to create a "family outing". Children may undertake an activity to please or impress their parents and peers.
- A parent will often buddy with their child who will have a reduced capacity to rescue their parent in an emergency.
- Diving equipment needs to be designed for children, including child-sized wetsuits, tanks, buoyancy compensators, regulator mouthpieces as well as masks, snorkels and fins.
- Children are often slim and weight belts may be poorly fitted and slip off leading to an uncontrolled ascent. Weights may need to be incorporated into the BCD.
- Children with a history of congenital heart disease who have existing right-to-left shunts or pulmonary hypertension would not be considered eligible to dive.

Consider the risk that the child is undertaking diving because of family or peer pressure.

Consider the risk of pulmonary barotrauma in a child with a history of bronchial hypersensitivity and asthma, (a possible, regular and major risk).

Consider the risk of poorly fitting equipment and ensure parents/diver centres are providing appropriately sized and designed equipment.

Consider the risk of 'executive dysfunction', especially in children diagnosed with attention deficit hyperactivity disorder (ADHD) and attention deficit disorder (ADD) causing a poor perception of risk, inappropriate acceptance of a high risk and inappropriate responses to danger.

**Some of these risks may be reduced by appropriate selection criteria for a child's diving program and training in classes specifically for the younger diver by instructors with experience in teaching children. When diving, the child should be accompanied and supervised by an experienced adult diver.**

Consider the risk of higher rates of barotrauma to the middle ear and sinuses (a possible, regular and minor risk).

**This risk may be reduced by ensuring the child can equalise their middle ears before each dive and is told to report any headache during or following a dive.**

Consider the risk of bubble formation in the epiphyses disrupting bone growth (a possible, rare and moderate risk).

**This risk may be reduced by limiting the depth and frequency of dives and always incorporating a safety stop.**

Consider the risk of hypothermia (a plausible, regular and moderate risk).

**This risk may be reduced by ensuring adequate thermal protection is worn and avoiding cold waters.**

Consider the risk of dehydration, (a plausible, regular and moderate risk).

**This risk may be reduced by ensuring the child is encouraged to drink adequate fluids before the dive.**

**We suggest that children be assessed for their fitness to dive from the age of 14 and upwards. Up to the age of 18, the input of their guardian is to be requested as well.**

## THE AGEING DIVER

- Diving became a popular sport in the 1960s and 1970s, so the population of ageing divers is expanding rapidly (the authors included). A few people learn to dive as a retirement recreation.
- Physical fitness, strength and agility all diminish with age. Specifically, lung compliance, maximum heart rate and oxygen uptake all fall with age.

- Many older divers do not dive regularly and become 'occasional' divers, e.g., when on a tropical holiday in warm waters.
- The incidence of chronic and degenerative diseases increases with age. Specifically, the incidence of coronary artery disease and diabetes increases with age.
- Diving fatality rates increase with age for both sexes. The higher relative risk for males progressively decreases until they are similar after the age of 60 (Denoble).
- Cardiac causes of death while diving dominates the over 45 years of age group (Caruso, Lippman).
- Some surveys show that many divers are diving with diseases such as ischaemic heart disease, hypertension, diabetes, PFOs, and asthma. Some follow the recommended guidelines but many, for fear of exclusion or insurance, do not (Lippman).
- Generally (but not dependably) wisdom and experience increase and risk-taking diminish with age.

Consider the risk of any known pre-existing pathology.

**This risk may be reduced by pre-dive and periodic medical examinations. Specifically consider physical fitness, comorbidities and mobility and strength (Strauss). 5 yearly examinations are suggested in divers >45 years and annually in divers 65 years or older or younger if they have ongoing or newly presented co-morbidities.**

Consider the risk of undiagnosed diabetes and possible ketoacidosis whilst diving (a possible, remote and major risk).

**This risk may be reduced by checking the fasting blood sugar and $HbA_{1c}$.**

Consider the risk of coronary artery disease first presenting during a dive (a possible, remote and major risk).

**This risk may be reduced by specifically asking about regular exercise and symptoms of ischaemic heart disease as well as performing an ECG and a formal cardiac risk assessment. Those people who have suspicious symptoms, an abnormal ECG or a risk >10% should have a cardiological review.**

**We advise older divers not to compete with the younger diver and to always buddy up with someone of similar age, fitness and interest.**

## FITNESS

- Physical fitness is one of the most important factors in diving safety. Fatigue is a very important contributing factor to panic. An unfit diver is more likely to get severe lactic acidosis from strenuous activity, hyperventilate and panic than a fit diver.
- Some studies suggest that nitrogen washout from the body may be related to their level of aerobic capacity; hence poor physical fitness may predispose to decompression illness (Ronning).
- Age, obesity, heavy smoking, and lack of regular exercise will all contribute to poor physical fitness.
- Fewer regular divers belong to clubs, own their equipment and dive regularly. Competition with other extreme sports reduces the commitment of people seeking thrills and adventure to one activity (Buzzacott).
- A minimum level of fitness equivalent to 7 METS has been suggested (Buzzacott) although a greater fitness level is preferred. This is equivalent to strenuous hiking, cycling 10-15mph on the flat, rowing, and skiing downhill.
- Fitness for physical activity is best tested by that activity itself, e.g., fitness to snow ski is poorly tested by one's fitness to play tennis. Diving demands some power and endurance in swimming, particularly finning. Many dive schools encourage divers to attain aquatic skills by being able to swim, unassisted by equipment, 200 metres in 5 minutes.

### Exercise programs for diving need to incorporate:

- power building e.g., swimming with a mask, snorkel and fins moderately fast to tire in 5 minutes.
- endurance building e.g., swimming with mask, snorkel and fins at a pace that can be maintained for at least 20 minutes.
- stretching after a gentle warm-up before exercise to limber up as well as after the exercise to expand the muscles.

In all divers who seem in poor physical condition, especially if they do not undertake regular aerobic exercise, we recommend a supervised swimming program before commencing diving.

It is important to match the exercise capabilities of buddies to prevent a diver from working beyond their capacity.

## SMOKING

- Traditionally 'pack-years' (one pack-year is the smoking of 20 cigarettes per day for one year) were used to quantify cigarette smoking habits as an aid to predict lung disease. However, the measurement of smoking using pack years is imprecise and raises concerns of inaccurate reporting and recall bias, especially for individuals whose smoking rate is low or fluctuating. The 'number of years smoking' may be a more sensitive, reliable, and efficient operational index of smoking exposure in predicting lung disease risk. Low-rate smokers demonstrated an increased risk of emphysema, despite a relatively low threshold of lifetime smoking exposure (6.4 pack-years) (Mathew).
- 50% of smokers eventually develop COPD (Marsh). Smoking also substantially increases the risk of cardiovascular disease including coronary heart disease, stroke, vascular disease, and aneurysms.
- Smoking causes an increase in mucus production in the nasopharynx and bronchial tree. These mucus plugs can block the Eustachian tube, preventing equalization of the middle ear and causing localised air trapping in the lungs.
- Smokers can have elevated levels of carboxyhaemoglobin, as high as 5%, which could limit exercise tolerance.
- When DCI occurs in recreational divers, smoking is a risk factor for increased severity of symptoms. It is not clear if smoking itself is a risk factor for getting DCI (Buch).
- Many individuals with less than 25% of lung tissue destroyed by emphysema are unaware of symptoms but will experience shortness of breath with mild exertion.

Consider the risk of increased pulmonary barotrauma of ascent caused by air trapping from mucus plugs or pulmonary infection (a possible, rare and major risk).

**This risk may be reduced by ensuring there is no active infection at the time of diving, all ascents are slow and controlled, and by stopping smoking.**

Consider the risk of increased middle ear and sinus barotrauma caused by mucus plugs in the upper respiratory tract (a plausible, regular and moderate risk).

**This risk may be reduced by education on middle ear equalization techniques and stopping smoking.**

Consider the risk of reduced exercise tolerance due to emphysematous lung damage (a plausible, remote and moderate risk).

**This risk may be reduced by early identification by a full spirometry assessment, regular aerobic exercise and by stopping smoking.**

Consider the risk of undetected coronary artery disease (CHD) causing sudden angina of effort during diving, especially if they have other risk factors for cardiac disease (a possible, remote and major risk).

**This risk may be reduced by specifically asking about regular exercise and symptoms of CHD. For anyone with any suspect symptom or several cardiac risk factors, an ECG and a formal cardiac risk assessment is recommended.**

# WEIGHT

A useful and simple assessment of weight is to calculate the Body Mass Index (BMI).

BMI = weight in kilograms/height in metres squared

Hence a diver 180 cm tall, 77 kg in weight has a BMI of 77 / 1.8 x 1.8 (3.24) = 23.8

In general, a BMI <19 = lean, 19-25 = normal, 26-30 = plump, 31-35 = obese, 36+ = morbid obesity.

**But beware, these ranges are only a guide since:**

1. there are significant racial variations and
2. a very muscular body will have a high BMI yet still be lean. It must be aligned with a sensible clinical assessment of body fat and waist circumference measurement.

# THE UNDERWEIGHT, BMI <19

- Low body weight may be pathological, e.g., eating disorder, malnutrition, malabsorption and malignancy.
- There is less body insulation and hypothermia may occur more readily.
- Equipment is usually designed for regular-sized individuals. Small sizes may be less readily available, especially in remote areas.
- Reduced body fat will make the body negatively buoyant. Less weight than normal may be required.

Consider the risk of underlying pathology or behaviour.

Consider the risk of hypothermia.

**This risk may be reduced by making the diver aware of their vulnerability, the dangers of hypothermia and advising the use of appropriately thick, well-fitting wetsuits with hoods or dry suits.**

# THE OVERWEIGHT, BMI >30

- Obese divers are over-represented in the diving death statistics. In one survey 38% of divers were obese compared to 25% of the local general population (Lippman).
- Obesity is commonly associated with reduced physical fitness.
- Obese people are at risk for developing many diseases, including hypertension, diabetes, ischaemic heart disease, stroke, sleep apnoea, dyslipidaemia, osteoarthritis and depression
- Obesity is associated with both higher bubble grades in Doppler ultrasound detection after scuba dives when compared to normal subjects and with an increased risk of decompression illness (Mendez).
- Equipment is usually designed for regular sizes. Extra-large sizes may be less readily available, especially in remote areas.Excess body fat is associated with increased buoyancy. Extra weights may be needed.

Consider the risk of reduced exercise tolerance causing fatigue.

**The risk may be reduced by regular exercise, especially a supervised swimming program completed before diving.**

Consider the risks of the co-morbidities commonly associated with obesity.

**This risk may be reduced by a full pre-dive medical assessment.**

Consider the risk of increased incidence of decompression illness.

**This risk may be reduced by limiting the depth and frequency of diving and always incorporating a safety stop.**

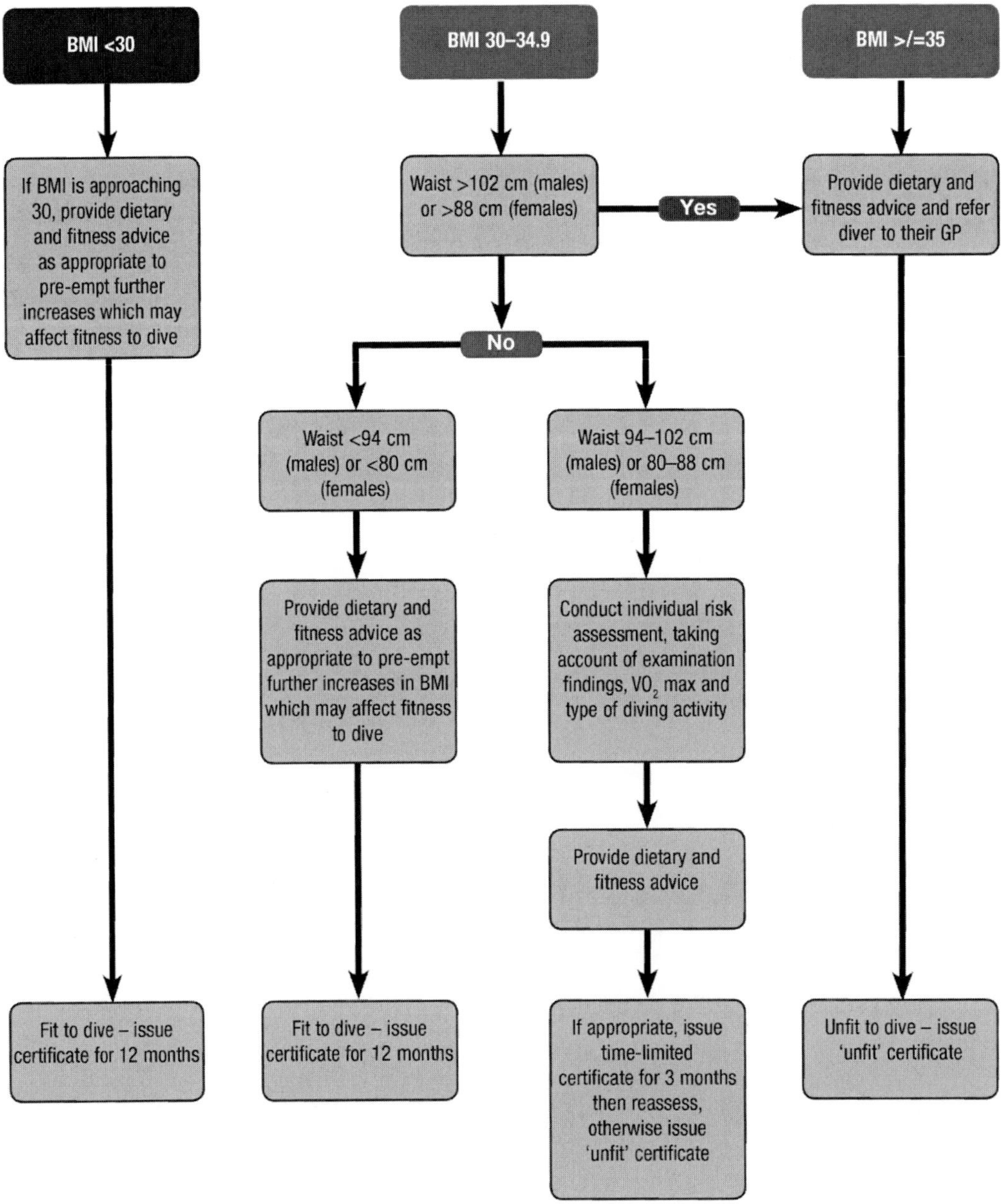


Management of elevated BMI. Reproduced with courtesy from HSE UK MA1 2015 version assessment form.

# FURTHER READING:


1. Buch DA, El Moalem H, Dovenbarger JA, Ugiccioni DM, Moon RE. Cigarette smoking and decompression illness severity: a retrospective study in recreational divers. Aviat Space Environ Med. 2003 Dec;74(12):1271-4. PMID: 14692470
2. Buwalda M, Querido AL, van Hulst RA. Children and diving, a guideline. Diving and Hyperbaric Medicine. 2020 December 20;50(4):399–404. doi: 10.28920/dhm50.4.399-404. PMID: 33325022.)
3. Buzzacott P, Pollock NW, Rosenberg M. Exercise intensity inferred from air consumption during recreational scuba diving. Diving and Hyperbaric Medicine. 2014 June;44(2):74-78.
4. Buzzacott P, Pikora T, Rosenberg M. Post-training dive inactivity in Western Australia. Diving and Hyperbaric Medicine. 2008; 38: 197-199.
5. Caruso J, Bove A A, Uguccioni D M, Ellis J E, Dovenbarger J A, Bennett P B. Recreational diving deaths associated with cardiovascular disease: Epidemiology and recommendations for pre-participation screening. Undersea Hyber Med 2001; 28(Supp): 75-6
6. Dembert M L, Keith J F. Evaluating the potential pediatric scuba diver. Am J Dis Child 1986; 140: 1135-41
7. Denoble PJ, Pollock NW, Vaithiyanathan P, Caruso JL, Dovenbarger JA, Vann RD. Scuba injury death rate among insured DAN members. Diving and Hyperbaric Medicine. 2008; 38: 182-188.
8. Divers Alert Network. Report on Decompression Illness and Diving Fatalities. 1998.
9. Dreyer S, Schneppendahl J, Moeller F, Koch A, Muth T, Schipke JD. An Updated Narrative Review on Ergometric Systems Applied to Date in Assessing Divers' Fitness. PMID: 34442180, PMCID: PMC8394438, DOI: 10.3390/healthcare9081044
10. Edmonds C. Scuba Kids. SPUMS J 1996; 26(3): 154-7
11. Egstrom G H. Are you ready to dive? Alert Diver May/June 1995: 30-5
12. JepsonN, RienksR, SmartD, BennettMH, MitchellSJ, Turner M. South Pacific Underwater Medicine Society guidelines for cardiovascular risk assessment of divers. Diving and Hyperbaric Medicine. 2020 September 30;50(3):273–277. doi: 10.28920/dhm50.3.273-277. PMID: 32957130
13. Krzyzak J, Korzeniewski K. Medical assessment of fitness to dive (Part I). Int Marit Health. 2021;72(1):36-45. doi: 10.5603/MH.2021.0005. PMID: 33829471
14. Krzyzak J, Korzeniewski K. Medical assessment of fitness to dive (Part I). Int Marit Health. 2021;72(2):115-120. doi: 10.5603/IMH.2021.0020. PMID: 34212351
15. Lippmann J, Taylor D McD, Stevenson C, Mitchell S. The demographics and diving behaviour of DAN Asia-Pacific members with and without pre-existing medical conditions. Diving and Hyperbaric Medicine. 2016 December;46(4):200-206.
16. Lippmann J, Lawrence CL, Fock A, Jamieson S, Harris R. Provisional report on diving-related fatalities in Australian waters in 2011. Diving and Hyperbaric Medicine. 2016 December;46 (4):207-240
17. Lippman J. A review of snorkelling and scuba diving fatalities in Queensland, Australia, 2000 to 2019. Diving Hyperb Med. 2022 Jun 30;52(2):108-118. doi: 10.28920/dhm52.2.108-118.
18. Martin L. Smoking and Diving – Is it really dangerous? Skin Diver Magazine, May 1996: 22Mathew AR, Bhatt SP, Colangelo LA, Allen NB, Jacobs Jr DR, Auer R, Dransfield MT, Hitsman B, Washko GR, Kalhan R. Life-Course Smoking Trajectories and Risk for Emphysema in Middle Age: The CARDIA Lung Study. Am J Respir Crit Care Med . 2019 Jan 15;199(2):237-240. doi: 10.1164/rccm.201808-1568LE.
19. Mendez-Dominguez N, Huchim-Lara O, Chin W, Carrillo-Arcio L, CamaraOKoyoc I, Cardenas-Daidai R, Dogre-Sansores O. Body mass index in association with decompression sickness events: cross-sectional study among small-scale fishermen-divers in southeast Mexico. Undersea Hyperb Med. Jul-Aug 2018;45(4):445-451. PMID: 30241124

20. Mitchell S. Junior open water divers and bubble-makers: Is age an issue? The Undersea Journal 2001; 74-6

21. Paton S. Fitness and the older diver. SPUMS J 1996; 26(4): 266-72

22. Pollock NW. Issues in the medical assessment of fitness to dive review. Int Marit Health. 2021;72(2):153. doi: 10.5603/IMH.2021.0030. PMID: 34212361

23. Rehman H V. Age and the cardiovascular system. Hosp Med 1999; 60(9): 645-9

24. Richardson D. Kids and Diving: The PADI Perspective. The Undersea Journal 2001; First Quarter: 8-13

25. Ronning P. Bolstad G. Does physical fitness influence the rate of nitrogen elimination in man? Collection of manuscripts for the XXIV Annual Scientific Meeting of the European Underwater and Baromedical Society, Gennser M (ed), Stockholm, Sweden. 1998: 117

26. Schwartz K. Age and diving. Alert Diver Sept/Oct 1996: 36-9

27. Strauss MB, Busch JA, Miller SS. Scuba in older-aged divers. Undersea Hyperb Med. Jan-Feb 2017;44(1):45-55. doi: 10.22462/1.2.2017.8.

28. PMID: 28768085

29. Taylor M. The young diver. Alert Diver (SEAP Edition) 2001; Jan-Mar:14-20

30. Viders H. Obesity and diving fitness. Alert Diver Sept/Oct 1998: 41-4

31. Williams N, Moore A, Woods M, Forman S. Audit of waist measurement methods during statutory diving medical assessments. Occup Med (Lond). 2021 Aug 20;kqab110. doi: 10.1093/occmed/kqab110. Online ahead of print. PMID: 34415343

32. Wingelaar TT, Bakker L, Nap FJ, van Ooij PJ, Endert EE, van Hulst R. Routine Chest X-Rays Are Inaccurate in Detecting Relevant Intrapulmonary Anomalies During Medical Assessments of Fitness to Dive. Front Physiol. 2021 Jan 6;11:613398. doi: 10.3389/fphys.2020.613398. eCollection 2020. PMID: 33488401, PMCID: PMC7816860

33. Winkler BE, Muth C-M, Tetzlaff . Should children dive with self-contained underwater breathing apparatus (SCUBA)? Acta Paediatr 2012 May;101(5):472-8. doi: 10.1111/j.1651-2227.2011.02589.x. PMID: 22212048

# Cardiovascular Disease

# 3

## POINTS TO PONDER:

**Cardiovascular disease is a common cause of death in divers. In one study of 877 diving deaths 14.8% were attributed to cardiovascular disease (Caruso).**

The cardiovascular system is commonly subjected to numerous stresses whilst scuba diving.

These include:

- **EXERCISE:** changes in exercise load can be sudden and unpredictable. Diving can involve strenuous and prolonged physical effort. It is not always possible to stop and rest. Dives often begin with a frantic swim to escape hostile surface conditions after sitting immobile in a small boat with no "warm-up" time possible.
- **ANXIETY:** this is common, especially in the novice but also in the experienced diver, causing increased heart rate and blood pressure.
- **PANIC:** severe anxiety is also common, even if usually only transitory. There may be a passive sympathetic discharge with a sudden, very high rise in pulse rate and blood pressure or a parasympathetic vagal response, with a slowing of the pulse and drop in blood pressure.
- **DIVING REFLEX:** a sudden immersion (especially of the face) into cold water may induce sudden bradycardia, an increase in blood pressure or even provoke dysrhythmia. Divers are partially protected by wearing a mask, until the mask is accidentally knocked and flooded, an event that can easily occur during a dive, especially on a jump or backward roll entry into the water.
- **HEAT:** diving in tropical waters combined with heavy exercise can raise body temperature, and reduce blood volume & blood pressure.
- **COLD:** cold will cause peripheral vasoconstriction and elevate blood pressure. It can occasionally provoke coronary artery spasm and angina. Cold may also provoke an immediate increase in oxygen consumption as a physiological response to generate more heat. Once cold stress is further increased, shivering will compound the demand. Cold will also cause a shift of blood from the skin and muscles into the central circulation and cause diuresis. After diving, on rewarming, restoration of the peripheral circulation may deplete the central circulation and cause hypotension (Doubt).
- **TOTAL BODY IMMERSION:** this will reduce the gravitational pooling of blood in the legs, causing a shift of 500-800 mls of blood into the central circulation. This central shift imposes a significant increase in cardiac load, with extrasystoles in

the early phase followed by diuresis. When combined with peripheral vasoconstriction, it is believed to explain rare episodes of immersion pulmonary oedema. Individuals with cardiac valvular disease, coronary artery disease, hypertension and blockade may be at higher risk. Total body immersion will also increase the drag of the body through the water (particularly when fully kitted up) and increase the energy requirements of swimming by up to 30% (Pendergast).

Sudden death in divers is usually caused by malignant dysrhythmias or asystole due to the above stressors and coronary artery disease. Such cardiac disease may be occult. The assessing doctor should always be suspicious of any diver with several risk factors for coronary artery disease. These include smoking, dyslipidaemia, hypertension, diabetes, male sex, obesity, age and family history of ischaemic heart disease.

## CORONARY ARTERY DISEASE

### Angina, Ischemic Heart Disease

- Diving frequently involves heavy, sudden exertion that will provoke angina and cause sudden disability. Ischaemic irritability of the myocardium may cause arrhythmias leading to sudden death.

Consider the risk of sudden anginal pain or even a myocardial infarction aggravated by sudden heavy exercise, cold and anxiety (a proven, regular and major risk).

Consider the risk of sudden death caused by arrhythmias aggravated by myocardial ischemia (a plausible, rare and major risk).

### The risks may be reduced if there are:

- no residual myocardial damage or pulmonary or neurological complications,
- no cardiac drugs are required for symptom control,
- a long symptom-free period (a minimum of a year is suggested),
- avoidance of risk factors for coronary artery disease,
- recent normal stress ECG and echocardiogram with a cardiological review,
- completion of a supervised exercise program and taking regular aerobic exercise,
- familiarity with the underwater environment,
- any proposed diving to be in sheltered (and preferably warm) waters,
- annual diving medical assessments.

**We would not recommend anyone with active symptoms of coronary artery disease to dive. The expertise of a cardiologist should be sought, also taking into consideration CT angiography and calcium score testing ± functional exercise testing.**

## MYOCARDIAL INFARCTION (MI)

### Heart Attack

- A history of MI reflects serious coronary artery disease. There will commonly be permanent myocardial damage.
- They may be on prophylactic medication, e.g., beta-blockers, or treatment of specific risk factors, e.g., antihypertensives or lipid-lowering drugs.

Consider the risk of sudden anginal pain or even another myocardial infarction aggravated by sudden heavy exercise, cold and anxiety (a proven, regular and major risk).

### The risk may be reduced if there are:

- no residual myocardial damage or pulmonary or neurological complications,
- no cardiac drugs are required for symptom control,
- a long symptom-free period (a minimum of a year is suggested),
- avoidance of risk factors for coronary artery disease,
- recent normal stress ECG and echocardiogram with a cardiological review,
- completion of a supervised exercise program and taking regular aerobic exercise,
- familiarity with the underwater environment,
- any proposed diving to be in sheltered (and preferably warm) waters,
- annual diving medical assessments.

Consider the risk of immersion pulmonary oedema (a plausible, rare and major risk).

**We would discourage anyone with a history of myocardial infarction to dive and only proceed if they were already experienced divers and had reduced the risk by following the suggested recommendations. If they were young with a history of isolated single vessel disease that had been corrected, one could be more liberal after careful assessment by a cardiologist, also taking into consideration CT angiography and calcium score testing ± functional exercise testing.**

## DYSRHYTHMIAS

- Immersion in water, especially cold water, may provoke dysrhythmias.
- Left ventricular hypertrophy is known to provoke various dysrhythmias and sudden death.

Consider the risk of any underlying medical condition.

Consider the risk of dysrhythmia compromising the cardiac output and exercise tolerance, leading to faintness, weakness and syncope.

Consider the risk of immersion-induced pulmonary oedema (a plausible, rare and major risk).

Consider the risk of a serious dysrhythmia causing sudden death (a possible, rare and major risk).

Consider the risk of dysrhythmia-provoking angina (a possible, rare and major risk).

**The risks will be dependent on the frequency and type of dysrhythmia. Many dysrhythmias are quite benign and disappear with an increased heart rate. Many are not.**

## SINUS BRADYCARDIA

- Common in young people, especially athletes, when it may be normal.
- Can be associated with cardiac disease and/or drugs, such as beta-blockers.

Consider the risk of sudden faintness, weakness, and even syncope with heavy exercise (a plausible, regular and moderate risk).

**This risk may be reduced by ensuring there is an appropriate exercise response.**

**We would refer anyone who did not increase their heart rate with exercise for a cardiological assessment.**

## ATRIAL ECTOPIC BEATS

- Frequently indicative of underlying cardiac pathology.
- May also have transient atrial flutter and fibrillation.
- Often associated with sick sinus syndrome, pulmonary hypertension and mitral/tricuspid insufficiency.

## FIRST DEGREE HEART BLOCK

### (Prolonged PR interval on the ECG)

- Can be caused by a high vagal tone in young adults.
- It is usually a significant sign of underlying cardiac disease.

Consider the risk that the diver has asymptomatic ischaemic heart disease and that diving could precipitate acute angina (a plausible, remote and major risk).

**This risk may be reduced by having a cardiological assessment and ensuring a normal stress ECG and echocardiogram.**

Consider the risk of immersion-induced pulmonary oedema (a possible, rare and major risk).

## SECOND DEGREE HEART BLOCK

### (Re-entrant tachycardia, Wolff-Parkinson-White Syndrome {WPW}, Lown-Ganong-Levine {LGL} syndrome)

- WPW is estimated to have an incidence of 0.1-0.3% of the population. Many people have a "concealed" aberrant accessory pathway when the ECG is normal. Even if someone has a secondary pathway, they may not conduct through it.
- WPW can be associated with hypertrophic cardiomyopathies.
- WPW can lead to atrial fibrillation and even ventricular fibrillation.

Consider the risk of a tachycardia occurring during a dive with associated reduced cardiac output, causing faintness, weakness and even syncope (a plausible, regular and moderate risk).

Consider the risk of aggravating an anginal pain during a palpitation occurring during diving (a possible, remote and major risk).

Consider the risk of precipitating ventricular fibrillation and sudden death (a possible, rare and major risk).

Consider the risk of immersion-induced pulmonary oedema (a possible, rare and major risk).

## SECOND DEGREE HEART BLOCK TREATED BY RADIO FREQUENCY CATHETER ABLATION

- Once successfully treated any associated risk is removed and the diver should be reassured.
- The success rate of the procedure is high but not guaranteed. Success can only be confirmed by electrophysiological and exercise studies.

## THIRD DEGREE HEART BLOCK / COMPLETE HEART BLOCK

- Commonly associated with ischaemic heart disease.

Consider the risk of an inadequate cardiac response to exercise with resultant faintness, weakness and syncope (a proven, regular, and major risk).

Consider the risk of immersion pulmonary oedema (a possible, rare and major risk).

**We would not recommend anyone with this condition to dive.**

## PAROXYSMAL SUPRAVENTRICULAR TACHYCARDIA PAROXYSMAL ATRIAL TACHYCARDIA

- In younger divers it is usually a benign condition, often aggravated by certain factors, such as caffeine, alcohol, nicotine, fatigue and hunger.
- In older divers, it can be associated with cardiac disease.

Consider the risk of aggravating an anginal pain during a palpitation occurring during diving (a plausible, remote and major risk).

Consider the risk of immersion pulmonary oedema (a possible, rare and major risk).

Consider the risk that the sudden tachycardia reduces cardiac output with weakness, faintness and occasionally syncope (a plausible, regular and moderate risk).

**The risks are minimized by avoiding any aggravating factors, having a cardiological assessment and waiting until symptoms have abated for a prolonged period before diving (six months is empirically suggested).**

## VENTRICULAR ECTOPICS (VE) EXTRASYSTOLES, PREMATURE BEATS

- Usually give no symptoms except the occasional "thump in the chest". Usually, disappear as the heart rate increases. May be aggravated by caffeine and nicotine.
- If they are frequent, complex and multifocal, persist or increase with exercise they may lead to ventricular tachycardias.

Consider the risk that they are not simple VEs.

**The risk may be reduced by checking their frequency and nature with a continuous 24-hour ECG and, if abnormal, having a cardiological assessment.**

## RIGHT BUNDLE BRANCH BLOCK (RBBB)

- Present in about 15% of the normal population. If a solitary finding, it is not commonly associated with cardiac disease.
- If present it should be investigated because of its association with interatrial septal abnormalities, particularly a patent foramen ovale (Bakalli, Gunes).

Consider the risk of associated coronary artery disease.

This risk may be reduced by ensuring there are no related symptoms. If present or there are significant risk factors for coronary artery disease, then a cardiological assessment should be arranged.

**If the diver has no aggravating factors, we would agree to diving.**

## INTRACARDIAC SHUNTS

- Venous gas emboli composed of inert gas (nitrogen/helium) commonly form in the circulation of sports divers on the ascent, most commonly peaking at 30-60 minutes post-dive.
- These bubbles are normally trapped and dissipated in the pulmonary vascular bed which acts as an effective filter.
- A diver who has an intracardiac or intrapulmonary shunt, which has a right-to-left flow (usually flow is left to right, but this pressure differential can be reversed on releasing a Valsalva manoeuvre or straining for example, commonly occurring post diving), may therefore be at risk of right to left shunting of venous gas emboli, causing a paradoxical arterial gas embolism and the subsequent neurological, vestibulocochlear or cutaneous symptoms.

**This will depend on the type of shunt:**

## ATRIAL SEPTAL DEFECT (ASD)

- With ASDs, even though the net flow is left to right, there are bi-directional flow phases during which right-to-left shunting of venous gas emboli may occur.
- Any right-to-left flow is increased by Valsalva manoeuvres, coughing and body immersion.
- ASDs may close spontaneously and are usually only closed surgically if they are symptomatic.

Consider the risk of right to left shunting of venous nitrogen bubbles causing an arterial gas embolism (a proven, remote and major risk).

**We do not recommend anyone with ASD to dive.**

## VENTRICULAR SEPTAL DEFECT (VSD)

- Flow through VSDs is always left to right, so there is no risk of arterial gas embolism, unless Eisenmenger syndrome has developed, resulting in a reversal of flow.
- Haemodynamically significant VSDs are usually surgically corrected.

Consider the risk of reduced exercise tolerance because of the left to right shunt (a possible, remote and moderate risk).

**If the diver has a history of good exercise tolerance, we recommend diving. If they do not do regular exercise, we ask for a cardiological assessment.**

## PATENT (PERSISTENT) FORAMEN OVALE (PFO)

- The foramen ovale is the bypass between the atria of the foetal heart to allow bypass of the pulmonary circulation, which should close at birth. Sometimes it fails to fully close, leaving a flap valve that can allow a right-to-left shunt, especially when the right atrial pressure is increased during a Valsalva manoeuvre, coughing or lifting.
- Its association with DCS has been well documented since the 1980s (Wilmshurst, Moon), but it has gained importance more recently due to prospective divers asking to be screened for its presence, both before any episode of DCS occurs, or after "unprovoked" DCS.
- Post-mortem studies show that about 30% of normal hearts have a probe-patent PFO. Confusion exists over the nomenclature used to describe PFOs (large/small, pencil or probe patent, grade 1, 2, or 3, significant, and so on) (Wilmshurst).
- Most PFOs are small and do not give rise to symptoms. Large PFOs predispose to cryptogenic stroke in young adults, as a result of paradoxical thromboembolism, and predispose to cutaneous and neurological (including vestibulocochlear) forms of decompression sickness (DCS) by paradoxical gas embolism, including strange presentations such as Anton

syndrome (Azzopardi). An association has been reported between migraine with aura and PFO (Wilmshurst).

- A PFO may not always be open. A sudden strain could force a previously lightly-fused PFO flap to tear open. There is also evidence for increasing patency of PFOs with advancing age, due to dehiscence of the flap (Wilmshurst).
- Diagnosing a PFO or ASD should be the remit of an experienced echocardiography operator, with the golden standard being trans-thoracic echocardiography with bubble contrast injection, coupled with provocative manoeuvres such as Valsalva and inspiratory sniff (Azzopardi).
- Trans-oesophageal echocardiography should be reserved for cases where the anatomy needs to be delineated in cases of PFO already being diagnosed and planned for PFO closure (PFOC) (Azzopardi).
- PFOs can now be surgically closed under radiological guidance, either with an umbrella device, such as the Amplatzer Occluder, or a novel procedure, such as the Noble Stitch (Madhkour).
- PFO closure (PFOC) is associated with documented complications, including thrombosis, dysrhythmias, device migration, and persistent shunt – complication rate variably ±8% (Scarff).

Consider the risk of increased incidence of serious cerebral, spinal & vestibulocochlear DCS (a proven, rare and major risk).

Consider the risk of increased incidence of cutaneous DCS (a proven, common and moderate risk).

Consider the risks of complications from PFO closure procedures.

**These risks may be reduced by limiting the depth to shallower than 15 metres and only doing a single dive per day, always using extended decompression according to DCIEM tables. Any activity that increases the pressure during or after diving e.g., forced Valsalva manoeuvres, should be avoided for at least 3 hours post-diving. These are termed conservative diving practices (CDPs).**

If a diver knows they have a large right-to-left shunt or one which spontaneously shunts on imaging, we warn them of the risks of serious subtypes of DCS, and strongly advise them not to dive. If they wish to accept the risk, we advise them to mitigate the risk by embracing the CDPs as delineated above.

After discussion with the diver and taking into consideration the merits of every case, we refer the diver to interventional cardiologists experienced in PFO closure and with a special interest in diving medicine.

**We do not recommend resumption of diving in divers who have undergone PFO closure until 3-6 months after the procedure, including imaging the device after a minimum of 3 months post-procedure to ensure closure of the shunt and exclude device migration, and only after stopping the anti-platelet medication 3-6 months post-shunt closure.**

## PERSISTENT DUCTUS ARTERIOSUS

- Small shunts can be asymptomatic. The shunt is always left to right and does not change with a Valsalva manoeuvre unless there is pulmonary hypertension.
- A large shunt is easily recognised by its continuous machinery murmur.
- All shunts are normally surgically closed to remove the risks of bacterial endocarditis.

Consider the risk of venous nitrogen bubbles traversing the pulmonary microcirculation causing an arterial gas embolism (if pulmonary hypertension coexists) (a possible, rare and moderate risk).

**To see a diver with an unrepaired ductus arteriosus would be rare. We would ask for a cardiological assessment.**

## REPAIRED DUCTUS ARTERIOSUS

Consider the risks of post-operative pleural adhesions.

## MURMURS

- Cardiac murmurs are commonly found at diving medicals and are usually benign. The diver frequently has no knowledge of it.
- It is important to take a full history of exercise tolerance and make a decision as to whether it is significant. If the cause is obscure or if there is any possibility it is an undiagnosed valve stenosis an echocardiogram should be obtained.

## PACEMAKERS

- The reason why a pacemaker has been fitted will normally define the risks for diving e.g., complete heart block or sick sinus syndrome.
- But there are benign reasons such as congenital heart block.
- The pressure specifications of pacemakers vary widely. Some are designed to withstand up to 4 ATA but some will not withstand 2 ATA pressure. One test to 6 ATA showed minor impressions from the underlying internal components with no influence on the function (Wonhas).
- Pacemakers vary in their response to exercise. It should be able to achieve 80% of the maximum pulse rate calculated for age (220 minus age in years).

Consider the risks of the underlying medical condition requiring the insertion of a pacemaker.

Consider the risks of the pressure limitations of the pacemaker.

Consider the risks of reduced exercise tolerance.

**We would strongly discourage anyone with a pacemaker to dive. If the reason for the pacemaker was benign and they were highly motivated, we would ask for a cardiological assessment. We would also confirm the pressure limitations and exercise response of their pacemaker with the manufacturer in writing.**

## IMPLANTABLE DEFIBRILLATORS

- Used to treat dysrhythmias such as ventricular tachycardia and fibrillation that lead to sudden death. There is a recurrence rate of dysrhythmia of 30-50% within 2 years.
- They contain air spaces and may be damaged by increases in pressure. Some brands are pressure-tested to shallow depths but this does not imply that they can be safely used whilst diving.

Consider the risk of the underlying cardiac pathology.

Consider the risk of the diver having dysrhythmia whilst diving and, even with a shock, reverting to normal rhythm becoming momentarily faint.

Consider the risk of the defibrillator being damaged and malfunctioning whilst under pressure.

**We would not recommend anyone with an implantable defibrillator to dive.**

# VALVULAR HEART DISEASE

## Regurgitation

- 25% of the population have some degree of aortic regurgitation and 30% have mitral regurgitation on colour doppler studies.
- Regurgitation can be increased if the systemic vascular resistance is increased by immersion and diving equipment such as a tight diving suit.
- Increases in central blood volume caused by immersion may aggregate the volume overload caused by major regurgitation to aggravate heart failure, especially when combined with an increased cardiac output caused by heavy exercise.

Consider the risk of aggravating acute heart failure and precipitating immersion pulmonary oedema (a plausible, remote and major risk).

**The risk may be reduced by ensuring there is no left ventricular hypertrophy or dysfunction on ECG or echocardiogram.**

**If the regurgitation is mild and the diver is doing regular exercise, we recommend diving. The diver should be advised to have annual medical checks to ensure that the regurgitation is not progressing. If the diver has more significant regurgitation, we would recommend an echocardiogram for further clarification before a cardiological assessment.**

# STENOSIS

- A stenotic aortic valve causes obstruction to the flow of blood through the heart, preventing a rapid increase in cardiac output in response to exercise and other stresses. It can present as a sudden death during exercise.
- A stenotic mitral valve can cause a rise in pulmonary venous pressure and lead to pulmonary oedema with exercise.

Consider the risk of provoking syncope, anginal pain or heart failure whilst exercising underwater (a proven, regular and major risk).

**We would not recommend anyone with valve stenosis to dive**

An overview of valvular disorders and their impact on diving follows:

| Valvular condition | Issues with diving |
|---|---|
| Aortic stenosis & idiopathic hypertrophic subaortic stenosis | Exercise syncope, sudden death, immersion pulmonary oedema (IPO) |
| Aortic regurgitation | None (heart failure if severe) |
| Mitral stenosis | Exercise induced pulmonary oedema |
| Mitral regurgitation | None (heart failure if severe) |
| Pulmonary stenosis | None (reduced exercise tolerance if severe) |
| Pulmonary regurgitation | Immersion pulmonary oedema (IPO) |
| Tricuspid stenosis | None (reduced exercise tolerance if severe) |
| Tricuspid regurgitation | None (heart failure if severe) |

| | |
|---|---|
| Atrial septal defect | Paradoxical arterial gas embolism |
| Ventricular septal defect | None if small |
| Patent ductus arteriosus | None (heart failure if severe) |
| Mitral valve prolapse | None (arrhythmias may accompany) |

Reproduced with permission from Bove & Davis, 4th edition, Saunders, 2003. V in Bove

## MITRAL VALVE PROLAPSE

### (Barlow's Syndrome, Floppy Mitral Valve Syndrome, "Click Murmur" Syndrome)

- Occurs in about 10% of the population.
- The amount of regurgitation is usually very small and of no clinical consequence. It is usually asymptomatic but can occasionally cause palpitations, chest pains and syncope.
- Treatment may include beta blockers.
- There is a rare incidence of sudden death because of prolonged Q-T interval syndrome.

Consider the risk of syncope aggravated by exercise whilst diving (a plausible, rare and major risk).

Consider the risk of sudden death (a possible, rare and major risk).

**If the diver is asymptomatic, we recommend diving. If they suffer any symptoms, we request a cardiological assessment.**

## CARDIAC TRANSPLANTATION

### Heart transplant

- The transplanted heart is denervated and does not always respond to exercise in a rapid or appropriate manner.
- The transplanted heart has a high incidence of development of coronary artery disease but because it is denervated, there is no warning pain.
- The diver is immunocompromised. The usual immunosuppressant drugs, azathioprine, prednisolone and cyclosporin have no specific adverse drug reactions (ADR) for diving but commonly cause nausea, general malaise, headache and dizziness. Toxic effects will result in neutropenia and thrombocytopenia, presenting as unexplained viral, fungal and bacterial infections, mouth ulcers, bruising and bleeding. Prednisone can predispose to oxygen toxicity, but this is usually only relevant to sports diving should the diver need recompression treatment.

Consider the risk of sudden death from ventricular tachycardia aggravated by heavy exercise in the denervated ischaemic heart (a possible, remote and major risk).

### This risk may be reduced if there are:

- no residual myocardial damage or pulmonary or neurological complications,
- no cardiac drugs are required for symptom control,
- a long symptom-free period (a minimum of a year is suggested),
- avoidance of risk factors for coronary artery disease,

- recent normal stress ECG and echocardiogram with a cardiological review,
- completion of a supervised exercise program and taking regular aerobic exercise,
- familiarity with the underwater environment,
- any proposed diving to be in sheltered (and preferably warm) waters,
- annual diving medical assessments.

Consider the risk of immersion pulmonary oedema (a possible, rare and major risk).

Consider the risk of adverse drug and toxic reactions from the immunosuppressive drugs.

Consider the risk of respiratory infections being caused by a contaminated regulator and/or buoyancy compensator.

**We would not recommend anyone with a history of cardiac transplantation to dive.**

## CARDIAC VALVE REPLACEMENT

- There may be more than one abnormal valve.
- If a metal or plastic valve has been inserted, the diver will be anticoagulated. Cardiac bypass surgery may cause pulmonary and neurological complications.
- Left atrial or ventricular enlargement may have occurred before surgery, with possible emboli occurring.
- Left heart valves occasionally fail, with catastrophic clinical results (approximately 1-2 per 1000 years).
- Some artificial valves cause the formation of micro-bubbles because of the cavitation caused. Whether these transient bubbles could act as bubble nuclei in supersaturated blood and so predispose to decompression illness (DCI) is unknown.

Consider the risks of anticoagulant drugs.

Consider the risk of sudden failure (a proven, rare and major risk).

Consider the risk of an increased incidence of DCI (a possible, rare and moderate risk).

**If the diver has a normal cardiac function, has suffered no pulmonary or neurological surgical complications and is not anticoagulated, we would recommend diving. If they are anticoagulated, we would strongly discourage them from diving.**

## CORONARY ARTERY BYPASS SURGERY

### Coronary Artery Angioplasty, Coronary Artery Stent

- Coronary artery surgery will relieve the most severe blockages but another coronary artery pathology will commonly exist. There may be significant pre-surgical cardiac damage.
- Coronary artery bypass surgery can cause neurological complications, particularly stroke (4.9%) and cognitive impairment (59%). There may be pleural adhesions.
- There is a high rate of re-stenosis after angioplasty (30%) and stenting (20%), usually within six months.

Consider the risk of any surgical complications.

Consider the risk of sudden anginal pain or even a myocardial infarction aggravated by sudden heavy exercise, cold and anxiety (a proven, regular and major risk).

Consider the risk of immersion-induced pulmonary oedema (a plausible, rare and major risk).

## These risks may be reduced if there are:

- no residual myocardial damage, pulmonary or neurological complications,
- no cardiac drugs are required for symptom control,
- a long symptom-free period (a minimum of a year is suggested),
- avoidance of risk factors for coronary artery disease,
- recent normal stress ECG and echocardiogram with a cardiological review,
- completion of a supervised exercise program and taking regular aerobic exercise,
- familiarity with the underwater environment,
- any proposed diving to be in sheltered (and preferably warm) waters,
- annual diving medical assessments.

**We would strongly discourage any diver with a history of coronary artery surgery to dive and only proceed if they were already experienced divers and had reduced the risk by following the suggested recommendations. If they were young with a history of isolated single vessel disease that had been corrected, one could be more liberal after careful assessment.**

# HYPERTENSION

- Blood pressure tends to rise with diving due to cold, anxiety, exercise and the fluid shift from the legs.
- Long-standing hypertension is associated with ischaemic heart disease (IHD), left ventricular hypertrophy (LVH), stroke, aortic aneurysm, peripheral vascular disease and pulmonary oedema.
- Unrecognised left ventricular hypertrophy is a common finding in autopsies of deceased divers. It is associated with an increased incidence of arrhythmias and sudden death (Buzzacott, Taylor).
- Antihypertensive drugs commonly alter the response of the heart rate and blood pressure to exercise, especially beta-blockers.

Consider the risk of associated coronary artery disease causing sudden anginal pain or myocardial infarction induced by heavy exercise (a proven, remote and major risk).

## This risk may be reduced by ensuring there are:

- good control of blood pressure,
- absence of end-organ damage especially left ventricular hypertrophy or dilation,
- prevention and/or treatment of risk factors for coronary artery disease,
- supervised exercise program.

Consider the risk of a stroke occurring whilst diving (a plausible, rare and major risk).

Consider the risk of immersion pulmonary oedema (a plausible, rare and major risk).

- This risk may be reduced by changing from beta-blocker medication.

Consider the risk of unrecognised LVF causing arrhythmias and sudden death.

**This risk may be minimised by performing an echocardiogram on any diver with a past or recent history of uncontrolled hypertension or signs of LVF on ECG (a proven, remote and major risk).**

Consider the risk of reduced exercise tolerance due to antihypertensive medication (a proven, regular and moderate risk).

**This risk may be reduced by checking for an appropriate cardiac response with exercise, especially in those divers who use beta blockers or who are on multiple drugs or who have high drug dosages.**

**We recommend diving if the blood pressure is well controlled, there is no sign of end-organ damage and there is a normal cardiac response to exercise. If they are physically unfit, we would recommend a supervised exercise program prior to diving.**

## PERIPHERAL VASCULAR DISEASE

- The presence of peripheral vascular disease is usually indicative of coexisting coronary and cerebral vascular disease.
- It is often associated with diabetes and heavy smoking.

Consider the risk of intermittent claudication aggravated by heavy finning causing sudden disability (a plausible, remote and moderate risk).

Consider the risk of sudden anginal pain aggravated by sudden heavy exercise (a plausible, remote and major risk).

**The risks may be reduced by ensuring the diver has completed a supervised exercise program, has a normal stress ECG and echocardiogram and avoids risk factors.**

**If a diver has symptoms or signs (such as carotid or femoral bruits) or absent pulses, we would very strongly discourage them from diving.**

## RAYNAUD'S PHENOMENON

- This spasmodic contraction of the digital arteries can be secondary to connective tissue disorder, obliterative arterial disease, occupations where the hands are exposed to vibration, cold agglutinins and cryoglobulins.
- Often aggravated by cold and emotion, it can result in thrombosis and ischaemic changes in the skin of the digits and nails.

Consider the risk of provoking severe ischaemic damage to the hands whilst diving (a plausible, remote and moderate risk).

**This risk may be reduced by using efficient thermal protection for the hands and feet and choosing to dive in warmer waters.**

**If Raynaud's phenomenon is easily aggravated by cold, we would strongly discourage diving. The use of thermal gloves should otherwise be encouraged.**

## DEEP VEIN THROMBOSIS (DVT)

- Aggravating factors include long-haul travel (air, rail, car and coach), previous thrombosis, hormonal therapy (including oral contraceptives), recent surgery, malignancy, pregnancy and certain haematological abnormalities (occurring in 3-5%of the population).
- The main danger of DVT is an embolus moving to the pulmonary circulation or heart causing sudden death or paralysis. There may be no warning symptoms.
- The mainstay of treatment is anti-coagulation to arrest the growth of the thrombus and prevent embolism. Anticoagulation is commonly continued for 3-6 months.

Consider the risk of leg exercise during finning causing the thrombus to embolise (a proven, regular and major risk).

Consider the risk of diving whilst being anticoagulated.

**Whilst the diver has symptoms or is on anticoagulants, we would not recommend diving.**

All divers on long-haul travel should take precautions to avoid DVT formation. This includes frequent short walks and flexing the ankles whilst sitting, avoiding dehydration by drinking plenty of fluids and avoiding alcohol. People at risk should wear support stockings to their lower legs to help prevent the pooling of blood.

## VARICOSE VEINS

- In themselves are not dangerous but if they are traumatised, they will bleed profusely, especially if they are engorged by the use of a tight short-legged wetsuit.
- Chronic venous insufficiency causes varicose eczema, especially in the skin of the lower shin. This is very vulnerable to chronic infection and ulceration.

Consider the risk of trauma to the lower limbs causing profuse bleeding or infection.

**This risk may be reduced by protecting the legs with a well-fitted long-legged wetsuit or elastic stocking.**

## FURTHER READING:


1. Allen M T, Shelley K S, Boquet A J Jr. A comparison of cardiovascular and autonomic adjustments to three types of cold stimulation tasks. Int J Pyschophysiol 1992; 13(1): 59-69
2. Azzopardi CP et al. Echocardiography – techniques and pitfalls whilst diagnosing persistent (patent) foramen ovale as a risk factor in divers with a history of decompression sickness. Diving Hyperb Med. 2021 March 31;51 (1):98-102. Doi: 10.28920/dhm51.1.98-102.
3. Azzopardi CP. Anton's syndrome as a presentation of decompression illness. Diving Hyperb Med. 2017 March;47(1):59-61.
4. Bakalli A, Koçinaj D, Georgievska-Ismail L, Bekteshi T, Pllana E, Sejdiu B. Right bundle branch block as a marker for interatrial septal abnormalities. Cardiol Young. 2012 Feb;22(1):18-25.
5. Balestra C, Germonpre P, Marroni A. Intrathoracic pressure changes after Valsalva strain and other manoeuvres: implications for divers with patent foramen ovale. Undersea Hyperb Med 1998; 25 (3):171-4
6. Bove A A. Risk of decompression sickness with patent foramen ovale. Undersea Hyperb Med 1998; 25(3): 175-8
7. Bove A A. Cardiovascular problems and diving. SPUMS J 1996; 26(3): 178-186
8. Buzzacott P, Edelson C, Bennett CM, Denoble PJ. Risk factors for cardiovascular diseases among active adult US scuba divers. Eur J Prev Cardiol. 2018 Sep;25(13):1406-1408. doi: 10.1177/2047487318790290. PMID: 30045634
9. Buzzacott P, Anderson G, Tillmans F, Grier JW, Denoble PJ. Incidence of cardiac arrhythmias and left ventricular hypertrophy in recreational scuba divers. Diving Hyperb Med. 2021 Jun 30;51(2):190-198. doi: 10.28920/dhm51.2.190-198. PMID: 34157735; PMCID: PMC8435355.
10. Caruso J L. Cardiovascular fitness and diving. Alert Diver July/Sept 1997: 10-5
11. Caruso J L, Bove A A, Uguccioni D M, Ellis J E, Dovenbarger J A, Bennett P B. Recreational diving deaths associated with cardiovascular disease: Epidemiology and recommendations for pre-participation screening. Undersea Hyber Med 2001; 28(Supp): 75-6
12. Doubt TJ. Cardiovascular &thermal responses to scuba diving. Med Sci Sports Exerc 1996; 28(5):581-586

13. Ewert P, Berger F, Daehnert I, Van Wees J, Gittermann M, Abdul-Khaliq H, Lange P E. Transcatheter closure of atrial septal defects without fluoroscopy: feasibility of a new method. Circulation 2000; 101(8): 847-9

14. Fitchet A, Fitzpatrick A P. Who needs an implantable defibrillator? Hosp Med 1999; 60(8): 578-83

15. Germonpre P. Persistent (patent) foramen ovale (PFO): implications for safe diving. Diving Hyperb Med 2015 Jun;45(2):73-4. PMID: 26165526

16. Grindley J, Mitchell S. Isolated pulmonary oedema associated with SCUBA diving. Emerg Med 1999; 11: 272-6

17. Gunes AE, Cimsit M. The prevalence of electrocardiogram abnormalities in professional divers. Diving and Hyperbaric Medicine. 2017 March;47(1):55-58.

18. Hampson N B, Dunsford R G. Pulmonary edema of scuba divers. Undersea Hyperb Med 1997; 24(1): 29-33

19. Ishikawa H, Matsushima M, Nagashima M, Osuga A. Screening of children with arrhythmias for arrhythmia development during diving and swimming – face immersion as a substitute for diving and exercise testing as a substitute for swimming. Jpn Circ J. 1992 Sep; 56 (9): 881-90

20. Jensen J H, Bonding P. Experimental pressure induced rupture of the tympanic membrane in man. Acta Otolaryngol Stockh 1993; 113(1): 62-7

21. Kilborn M J. Atrial Fibrillation. Med J Aust 1999; 170(10): 498-504

22. Kluger M. Atrial fibrillation presenting as decompression illness. SPUMS J 1993; 23(4):186-188

23. Langdon P. Patent foramen ovale in underwater medicine. SPUMS J 1996; 26(3): 186191

24. Madden D, Ljubkovic M, Dujic Z. Intrapulmonary shunt and SCUBA diving: another risk factor? Echocardiography 2015 Feb;32 Suppl 3:S205-10. doi: 10.1111/echo.12815. PMID: 25693625

25. Madhkour R, Wahl A, Praz F, Meier B. Amplatzer patent foramen ovale occluder: safety and efficacy. Expert Rev Med Devices 2019 Mar;16(3):173-182. doi: 10.1080/17434440.2019.1581060. Epub 2019 Feb 18. PMID: 30741039

26. Marchitto N, Iannarelli N, Paparello PT, Cioeta E, Parisi F, Pirrone S, Raimondi G. Cardiovascular risk in scuba divers. J Sports Med Phys Fitness. 2019 Oct;59(10):1779-1782. doi: 10.23736/S0022-4707.19.09358-7. PMID: 31311237

27. Moon R E, Byrne J C, Webb-Peploe M M. Patent foramen ovale and decompression sickness in divers. Lancet 1989; i: 513-4

28. Pendergast D R, Tedesco M, Nawrocki D M, Fisher N M. Energetics of underwater swimming with scuba. Med Sci Sports Exerc 1996; 28(5): 573-80

29. Pristipino C et al. European position paper on the management of patients with patent foramen ovale. Part II - Decompression sickness, migraine, arterial deoxygenation syndromes and select high-risk clinical conditions. EuroIntervention 2021; 16.

30. Scarff CW, Lippmann J, Fock A. A review of diving practices and outcomes following the diagnosis of a persistent (patent) foramen ovale in compressed air divers with a documented episode of decompression sickness. Diving Hyperb Med 2020 Dec 20;50(4):363-369. doi: 10.28920/dhm50.4.363-369. PMID: 33325017

31. Schagatay E, Andersson J, Holm B. The triggering of the human diving response. Collection of manuscripts for the XXIV Annual Scientific Meeting of the European Underwater and Baromedical Society. Gennser M. (ed), Stockholm, Sweden Aug 1998: 88-91

32. Smart D, Mitchell S, Wilmshurst PT, Turner M, Banham N. Diving Hyperb Med 2015 Jun;45(2):129-31. Joint position statement on persistent foramen ovale (PFO) and diving. South Pacific Underwater Medicine Society (SPUMS) and the United Kingdom Sports Diving Medical Committee (UKSDMC). PMID: 26165538

33. Van den Eede M, van Berendoncks A, De Wolfe D, De Maever C, Van den Eede H, Germonpre P. Percutaneous closure of patent foramen ovale for the secondary prevention of decompression illness in sports divers: mind the gap. Undersea Hyperb Med 2019 Sep - Dec - Fourth Quarter;46(5):625-632. PMID: 31683360

34. Taylor SE, Taylor DM, Pisasale D, Booth K, Lippmann J. Regular medication use by active scuba divers with a declared comorbid medical condition and victims of scuba and snorkelling-related fatalities. Diving Hyperb Med. 2021 Sep 30;51(3):264-270. doi: 10.28920/dhm51.3.264-270. PMID:

35. Wilmshurst PT, Ellis BG, Jenkins BS. Paradoxical gas embolism in a scuba diver with an atrial septal defect. Br Med J (Clin Res Ed). 1986;293(6557):1277. PMID: 3096463. PMCID: PMC1342110.

36. Wilmhurst P T, Nuri M, Webb-Peploe N M. Cold induced pulmonary oedema in scuba divers and swimmers and subsequent development of hypertension. Lancet 1989; 1: 62-65

37. Wilmshurst P, Treacher D F, Crowther A, Smith S E. Effects of patent foramen ovale on arterial saturation during exercise and on cardiovascular responses to deep breathing, Valsalva manoeuvre and passive tilt: relation to history of decompression illness in divers. Brit Heart J 1994; 71: 229-31

38. Wilmshurst P T, Nightingale S, Walsh K P, Morrison W L. Effect on migraine of closure of cardiac right-to-left shunts to prevent recurrence of decompression illness or stroke or for haemodynamic reasons. Lancet 2000; 356: 1648-51

39. Wilmshurst PT, Morrison LW, Walsh KP. Comparison of the size of persistent foramen ovale and atrial septal defects in divers with shunt-related decompression illness and in the general population. Diving Hyperb Med 2015 Jun;45(2):89-93. PMID: 26165530

40. Wilmshurst PT. The role of persistent foramen ovale and other shunts in decompression illness. Diving Hyperb Med 2015 Jun;45(2):98-104. PMID: 26165532

41. Wilmshurst PT. Risk mitigation in divers with persistent (patent) foramen ovale. Diving Hyperb Med 2019 Jun 30;49(2):77-78. doi: 10.28920/dhm49.2.77-78. PMID: 31177512 PMCID: PMC6704006

42. Wonhas C, Wnohas-Thiele H. Implanted Cardiac Defibrillator (ICD) and Pacemaker (PM) after long time hyperbaric oxygen therapy (HBO). Undersea Hyper Med 2000; 27(Supp): 32

43. Zimmerman D L, Loken R G, Hamilton R C. The diving reflex: bradycardia during cold ocular irrigation (letter; comment). Can J Anaesth 1994; 42(9): 875-6

# Connective Tissue and Rheumatic Diseases

# 4

## POINTS TO PONDER

**This section includes a spectrum of diseases where often the boundaries of diagnosis widely overlap. The spectrum has many common characteristics.**

- They are multi-system diseases, which often fluctuate with relapses and remissions.
- They commonly have an insidious onset and there may be a long delay between the onset of symptoms and diagnosis.
- Common symptom is fatigue and general malaise.
- Patients are commonly on medication, which may have significant adverse drug reactions, e.g., NSAIDS, prednisone, methotrexate, other immunosuppressant agents and various analgesics. Occasionally antidepressants are prescribed.
- Anyone with advanced disease will have multi-organ involvement (such as joints, bone, skin, lungs and heart) posing potential major risks. Diving would not be recommended. Approximately 5-10% of patients are in remission. All such need to be assessed by a rheumatologist with respect to the risks related to their illness and medication.

## ANKYLOSIS SPONDYLITIS

### Sacro-ileitis

- Extra-articular features include recurrent iritis, aortic regurgitation, cardiac conduction defects, apical pulmonary fibrosis, osteoporosis, and myelopathy associated with atlantoaxial subluxation.
- A limitation of ventilation is a common occurrence through the involvement of the costovertebral joints.
- Intrinsic lung disease affects about 1% of cases.

Consider the risk of a cardiac complication, especially dysrhythmias.

**This risk may be reduced by a cardiological assessment prior to diving.**

Consider the risk of any associated pulmonary complication, especially apical fibrosis.

**This risk may be reduced by a chest X-ray prior to diving to exclude fibrosis.**

Consider the risk of a reduction of ventilatory capacity, limiting exercise tolerance.

**This risk may be reduced by a full spirometric assessment prior to diving.**

Consider the risk of reduced spinal mobility and reduced agility.

**If lung function is normal and there are no cardiac complications, we recommend diving.**

## ARTHRITIS (OSTEOARTHRITIS, GOUT ARTHROPATHY)

- The major feature is joint pains, often associated with joint swelling and tenderness.
- Mobility and agility may both be compromised.
- It has been suggested that arthritic joints could be more susceptible to decompression illness.

Consider the risk of reduced mobility and agility leading to falls when kitting up and entering and exiting sites,(a plausible, remote and moderate risk).

**This risk may be reduced by choosing diving sites and times where access and conditions are stable.**

Consider the risk of an increased incidence of decompression illness (a possible, rare and moderate risk).

**This risk may be reduced by limiting the depth and frequency of diving and always including a safety stop.**

Consider the risk of confusing joint pains following a dive due to "arthritis with decompression illness (a possible, rare and moderate risk).

**If the diver has reasonable mobility, we warn them of the common problems encountered with mobility whilst diving and recommend diving.**

## RHEUMATOID ARTHRITIS / SERO-NEGATIVE ARTHRITIS

- This is not just arthritis but a systemic disease where the joints usually give most of the symptoms.
- The hands are commonly involved with weakness of grip.
- Involvement of the cervical spine may cause subluxation of the atlantoaxial spine.
- Lung involvement is uncommon but may include asymptomatic pleural effusion, pulmonary fibrosis and rheumatoid nodules in the lung parenchyma.
- Constrictive pericarditis can occur with few if any, symptoms until prolonged exercise demands a higher cardiac output.
- Muscle wasting may cause significant weakness.
- "Rheumatoid ear" has been described with related stiffness of the tympanic membrane and ossicular chain which theoretically could predispose to aural barotrauma.

Consider the risk of fatigue and reduced general body strength.

Consider the risk of aural barotrauma from "rheumatoid ear" (a possible, rare and minor to moderate risk).

Consider the risk of asymptomatic pulmonary involvement reducing exercise tolerance and predisposing to pulmonary barotrauma.

**This risk may be reduced by confirming lung integrity with a chest X-ray prior to diving. Only the diver with mild uncomplicated disease should dive.**

## SYSTEMIC LUPUS ERYTHEMATOSUS (SLE)

- This generalised inflammatory disease affects many organs by immune complexes being deposited in the tissues. Many patients have very mild disease that should not impact diving.
- Symptoms may include Raynaud's phenomena, pericarditis, fibrosing alveolitis, "shrinking lung syndrome", as well as avascular necrosis of the femoral head.
- Pleuro-pulmonary disease is present in 50% of patients, the common manifestations being pleuritis and atelectasis.

Consider the risk of pleural pulmonary complications predisposing to pulmonary barotrauma.

Consider the risk of aggravating Raynaud's phenomenon.

Consider the risk of easy fatigue because of malaise and poor physical fitness.

**Only the diver with mild uncomplicated disease should dive.**

## SCLERODERMA

### Progressive systemic sclerosis, CRST or CREST syndromes

- Severe Raynaud's phenomena are usually the presenting symptom.
- Pulmonary fibrosis occurs in most cases.
- Loss of lower oesophagus peristalsis predisposes to gastric reflux.
- Other complications include cardiomyopathy, heart block and aortic valve lesions.
- Treatment may include a wide range of medications.

Consider the risk of easy fatigue because of malaise and poor physical fitness.

Consider the risk of aggravating Raynaud's phenomena.

Consider the risk of pulmonary fibrosis predisposing to pulmonary barotrauma.

Consider the risk of gastric reflux causing acute oesophageal spasm whilst diving in an upside-down position.

**Only the diver with mild uncomplicated disease should dive.**

## VASCULITIS

### Polyarteritis Nodosa, Wegener's Granulomatosis

- This group of conditions is characterised by focal and segmental inflammation of blood vessels.
- Pathological changes include aneurysm formation, vessel wall rupture and thrombosis resulting in local ischaemia or infarction.
- Symptoms may mimic and be confused with decompression illness (DCI).
- Decompression illness may even be aggravated in tissues already haemodynamically compromised.

- The coronary arteries can be involved with risk of infarction or sudden death. Pulmonary infiltrates and asthma occur.
- CNS involvement includes polyneuropathy, convulsions, hemiplegia, and psychoses.
- Renal involvement causes hypertension, proteinuria, renal failure and intra-renal aneurysms.

Consider the risk of possible hypertension and coronary artery involvement causing angina or myocardial infarction.

Consider the risk of pulmonary involvement causing pulmonary barotrauma. Consider the risk of symptoms being confused with DCI.

**Only the diver with mild uncomplicated disease should dive.**

## FURTHER READING:

1. Benton P J, Smith R W. Vasculitis masquerading as neurological decompression illness. Undersea Hyperb Med 1996; 23(3): 189-91
2. Paul R A, Helle M J, Tarssanen. Sudden death as sole symptom of coronary arteritis. An Med 1990; 22: 161-2
3. Rowe-Jones J M, Macallan D C, Sorooshian M. Polyarteritis nodosa presenting as bilateral sudden onset cochlea- vestibular failure in a young woman. J Laryngol Otol 1990; 104: 562-4

# Dental Issues

# 5

## POINTS TO PONDER

The mouth and teeth are important body parts in scuba diving because they hold the regulator that provides the air supply.

Faults in the teeth or dental fillings may be subject to barotrauma of descent and ascent.

## CARIES

- A carious tooth containing a cavity can implode as the wall of the cavity collapses on descent.
- Alternatively, a carious cavity behind a cracked filling may slowly allow air to enter on descent but on ascent explode as the air is unable to escape quickly.

Consider the risk of dental barotrauma (or barodontalgia) (a proven, remote and minor risk).

**This risk may be reduced by regular dental check-ups.**

## CROWNS

- Studies have shown that the retention of full cast crowns to extracted teeth may be reduced by up to 66% by repeated diving.
- The type of cement and post (if used) was significant, with fibre-reinforced posts and resin cement being found superior (Musajo), (Lyons), (Mitoy), (Safia).

Consider the risk of crowns being weakened and more easily dislodged.

**This risk may be reduced by using resin cement when applying crowns.**

## DENTAL FILLINGS

- Cracked fillings can allow gas to seep behind the filling on descent. Subsequent rapid expansion can cause a toothache or even for the filling to be pushed out of the tooth.
- Incomplete root canal treatment with temporary fillings may contain possible tiny air spaces that can also cause toothache.
- Underwater welding can cause a metallic taste and erosion of metal fillings.

Consider the risk of dental barotrauma (a proven, remote and minor risk).

**This risk may be reduced by regular dental check-ups.**

## DENTAL EXTRACTIONS

- Whilst diving, the pressured air can track through the broken oral mucosa and into the submucosal tissues. On the ascent, as the gas expands, it may not exit through the wound but track in the submucosal plane to cause submucosal emphysema.
- There are many pathogens in seawater with the subsequent risk of infection of the tooth socket.

Consider the risk of submucosal emphysema (a plausible, remote and minor risk).

**This risk may be reduced by allowing sufficient time to allow full healing of the oral mucosa before diving.**

Consider the risk of infection of the tooth socket.

**This risk may be reduced by allowing sufficient time to allow full healing of the oral mucosa before diving.**

## DENTURES

- The regulator needs to be comfortable and secure in the mouth so any denture must be well-fitted.
- Partial dentures may become dislodged during diving when it is awkward to refit them.

Consider the risk of dentures becoming dislodged whilst diving.

**This risk may be reduced by ensuring that dentures are tight-fitting and partial dentures are clasped.**

## MOUTH ULCERS

- There are many causes of mouth ulcers, e.g., infective, aphthous, malignant, and systemic, some of which have serious implications for diving.
- Holding the regulator in the mouth for extended periods may aggravate the ulceration causing severe local pain and discomfort.
- If the cause of the ulcer is infective, e.g., herpetic, sterilization of the regulator before use by other divers is important.

Consider the risks of any underlying medical condition.

Consider the risk of severe oral pain during the dive from irritation of the ulcers by the regulator.

## ORTHODONTIC APPLIANCES

### Braces

Hard rubber regulator mouthpieces may abrade the appliances. It is recommended to use soft silicone rubber mouthpieces or even have custom-made, moulded mouthpieces.

## PERIODONTAL DISEASE

In advanced disease, gum retraction and loose teeth may occur.

# TONGUE BOLTS

## Studs

- These are becoming popular and seem to have no harmful effects whilst diving.
- The bolt should be checked for tightness before diving.

# FURTHER READING:


1. Elnaz S, Reza F, Amir RB. Impact of various pressures on fracture resistance and microleakage of amalgam and composite restorations. Diving Hyperb Med 2018 Sep 30;48(3):168-172.
2. Gougeon K, Yasukawa K, Baudet A. Barodontalgia and Dental Barotrauma Among Scuba Divers. Aerosp Med Hum Perform. 2022 May 1;93(5):539. doi: 10.3357/AMHP.6045.2022. PMID: 35551726
3. Hammond J. Orthodontic treatment and diving. Br J Orthopod 1997; 24(4): 346-7
4. Hobson R S, Newton J P. Dental evaluation of scuba diving mouthpieces using a subject assessment index and radiological analysis of jaw position. Br J Sports Med 2001; 35: 84-8
5. Jones T. Popping Teeth. SSI Dive Business International. 1999 3rd Quarter: 24-25
6. Kieser J, Holborow D. The prevention and management of oral barotrauma. N Z Dent J 1997; 93(4): 114-6
7. Lyons K M, Rodda J C, Hood J A. Barodontalgia: a review and the influence of simulated diving on microleakage and on the retention of full cast crowns. Mil Med 1999; 164(3): 221-227
8. Mitov G, Draenert F, Schumann P, Stotzer M, von See C. The influence of pressure changes on the retentive force and coronal microleakage of different types of posts in endodontically treated teeth during simulated dives. Diving Hyperb Med . 2016 Dec;46(4):247-252.f
9. Musajo F, Passi P, Girardello G B, Rusca F. The influence of environmental pressure on retentiveness of prosthetic crowns: an experimental study. Quintessence Int 1992; 23(5): 367-9
10. Nakdimon I, Zadik Y. Barodontalgia Among Aircrew and Divers. Aerosp Med Hum Perform. 2019 Feb 1;90(2):128-131. doi: 10.3357/AMHP.5183.2019. PMID: 30670123
11. Pooria S, Babak F, Reza F. The effects of pressure in vitro on three methods of root canal obturation. Diving Hyperb Med 2019 Mar 31;49(1):16-20.

# Dermatological Issues

# 6

## POINTS TO PONDER

- The integrity of the skin can be compromised by the diving environment. Prolonged immersion and high humidity will soften the stratum corneum causing desquamation and altering the surface pH allowing a change in the skin's bacterial and fungal flora.
- The skin is also commonly subject to numerous other insults whilst diving.
  - » Chafing, especially by wet swimwear, wet wetsuits, masks and fins.
  - » Minor abrasions and lacerations from equipment, e.g., rubbing from fins, the boating environment, e.g., stubbing toes on boats, and the marine environment, e.g., coral cuts.
  - » Stings from marine animals and plants.
  - » Urine irritation from urinating in wetsuits whilst diving due to the induced diuresis whilst underwater, small bladder capacity or as a warming technique.
  - » Salt, which is hydrophilic and abrasive.
- Seawater contains many unusual and hardy organisms which can infect any break in the skin, especially if it is implanted by trauma into skin softened by immersion. Such organisms include Vibrio, Aeromonas, Mycobacterium, Erysipelothrix and Protothecosis (Qureshi).
- Dry suit squeeze can subject the skin to negative pressures.
- Compressed air over broken skin can track into the subcutaneous layer and cause swelling and pain.

## BURNS AND OPEN WOUNDS

- Prolonged immersion in water will predispose to infection and delay healing.

Consider the risk of the burn or wound becoming infected.

**This risk may be reduced if the burn or wound is small, protected with a waterproof dressing during the dive and the immersion period is limited by shortening the dive time and restricting the number of dives a day.**

# COLD URTICARIA

## Acquired cold urticarial syndrome (ACU)

- This syndrome can cause a person who is suddenly exposed to cold to develop a rash. They may become hypotensive, and even lose consciousness.
- One study found 5.7% of their urticaria patients had cold urticaria, mainly young women.
- 77% of people with cold urticaria break out in a generalized urticarial rash and 44% had "shock-like reactions" with dizziness and fainting fits.
- The commonest cause of cold urticaria is aquatic activity.

Consider the risk of sudden faintness and even syncope whilst underwater (a plausible, remote and major risk).

**This risk may be reduced by pre-treatment with non-sedating antihistamines.**

**We would not recommend anyone who experiences dizziness or fainting, to dive.**

# CERCARIAL DERMATITIS

## Swimmer's itch

- Cercarial dermatitis is caused by mammalian and avian schistosomes of the family Schistosomatidae. Freshwater species of Schistosoma, marine species of Austrobilharzia and Ornithobilharzia, and freshwater/marine species of Trichobilharzia, Gigantobilharzia, Anserobilharzia, Allobilharzia, and Dendritobilharzia have all been implicated.
- Birds and rodents, the definitive hosts, excrete schistosome ova into the water that mature into free-swimming miracidiae. These miracidiae infect snails and transform into cercaria larvae that penetrate the human stratum corneum.
- Humans represent the final hosts as the larvae eventually die within the skin. The immunogenic enzymes of the cercariae result in sensitization 2 weeks after the first contact. Subsequent exposure results in lesions within hours (Sridhar).

# CORAL DERMATITIS

- Dermatitis can develop after physical contact with one of many coral species that produce toxic mucinous exudate and nematocysts.
- The ensuing rash appears over a period of minutes to days, possibly due to a hypersensitivity reaction.
- Such contact may lead to abrasions and deposition of a mucinous exudate and nematocysts.
- Washing the affected skin with vinegar or applying cold packs may help remove or neutralize unfired nematocysts.
- However, if a rash consistent with coral dermatitis develops, the treatment of choice is a topical steroid.
- Patients should be counselled to seek further medical attention if the initial rash worsens despite steroid therapy or does not resolve within 2 weeks, if systemic symptoms develop, or if a delayed granulomatous rash appears (Ceponis).

# CORAL CUTS

- The smallest scratch from coral or any marine organism can readily become infected. This is even worse with diving for the prolonged immersion softens and macerates the skin reducing its natural defences.
- Foreign body reactions from implanted fragments may occur.

**All divers should be warned of the dangers of infection from any abrasion and informed of the correct treatment, namely:**

- Remove all foreign bodies from the wound and clean it thoroughly by scrubbing it in warm soapy water. (It is advisable for all divers to carry a soft toothbrush for this purpose)
- Clean the wound with an antiseptic solution, e.g., chlorhexidine 0.1% or povidone-iodine 10%.
- Apply a thin smear of broad-spectrum antibiotic.

**All divers should be advised to ensure their tetanus vaccination is current.**

## DIVERS GREEN HAIR

- Occasionally divers with blonde hair, especially those with dyed or bleached blonde hair, note a greenish discolouration after using swimming pools recently treated with a copper algaecide solution.

## ECZEMA

### Dermatitis

- Prolonged immersion in water will cause softening of the skin and maceration predisposing pre-existing dermatitis to skin infection.

Consider the risk of provoking an infection in an area of chronic dermatitis, especially where a large surface area is involved (a plausible, remote and minor risk).

### This risk may be reduced by:

- Avoiding diving whilst large areas of dermatitis are acutely inflamed.
- After diving, the skin should immediately be rinsed with clean fresh water followed by thorough drying and application of a moisturizing cream.

**Should dermatitis become infected, diving should be discontinued and the use of antibiotics considered.**

## ECZEMA OF THE OUTER EAR CANAL

- Eczema or seborrheic dermatitis of the outer ear canal can cause pain and discomfort. Moreover, the retained desquamated skin makes it very prone to recurrent otitis externa.

Consider the risk of recurrent otitis externa (a proven, regular and minor risk).

**This risk may be reduced by having the patency of the ear canals checked before diving and following recommended ear care. See Appendix B.**

## CONTACT ALLERGIC ECZEMA

- Vulcanized rubbers are a common allergy and use to cause problems with masks, snorkels and fins. Neoprene, the isomer of chloroprene, is much safer but some of the added antioxidants, accelerants and the glue with which it is attached to the lining may be allergenic. Common allergens include diethyl thiourea, mercatobenzothiazole, thiuram, dithiocarbamates, paraphenylendiamine, formaldehyde, urea-formaldehyde resins, isopropyl-phenyl-parapheynlenediamine-thiourea (Okawa, Bergendorff).
- Most masks are now made from silicone rubber.
- Any history of rubber allergy, e.g., to rubber bands, rubber sports equipment, and escalator rails should be a warning of possible problems with rubber diving equipment (Weinberger).

## FACIAL CUTS

- Recent lacerations of the skin on the face within the mask area, especially of the eyebrows, may allow air to enter and track along the subcutaneous tissues to form subcutaneous emphysema on ascent.

## HERPES SIMPLEX ON THE FACE

### Cold sores

- Herpes simplex on the lips can be irritated by the regulator mouthpiece and become infected.
- Herpes simplex on the face can be irritated by the mask and become infected.
- It can be aggravated by sunlight and worsen during a dive trip.

## PHOTOSENSITIVITY OF THE SKIN

- Many drugs increase the sensitivity of the skin to sunlight, which is then prone to sunburn e.g., tetracyclines, tretinoin, naproxen, and furosemide.

## SCARRING ON THE FACE

- Severe scarring of the face, particularly from burns can interfere with the seal of the mask. Finding a mask that seals is essential for enjoyable diving.

## SKIN INFECTIONS

### Bacterial e.g. Impetigo
### Fungal e.g. Tinea

- Prolonged immersion, humid environment and chafing will all aggravate existing skin infections and delay healing.

Consider the risks of aggravating the infection.

**Tinea cruris ("Jock itch") especially is aggravated by the chafing of wet swimmers and they should be removed as soon as possible after a dive and replaced by dry, non-chafing clothes. Tinea pedis (athletes' foot) is also common and prone to infection. Special care should be made to dry the feet after diving and keep them dry between dives.**

**Divers prone to tinea may use an anti-fungal cream prophylactically when doing multiple dives.**

## SUNBURN

- This is one of the commonest problems that spoils a diving holiday, especially in the tropics.

### Any diver going to a sunny climate should be advised to avoid sunburn. This should include:

- Wearing a broad-brimmed hat and long-sleeved shirts whenever in the sun.
- Applying a waterproof 50+ sunscreen several times a day, the first time being before sun exposure when the skin is still dry.
- Only exposing the skin to short periods of sunlight (initially 10-20 minutes), especially during the peak ultra-violet periods of the day, 10 am – 2 pm.

# FURTHER READING:


1. Balestrero S, Cozzani E, Ghiglotti G, Guarrera M. Allergic contact dermatitis from a wetsuit. J Eur Dermato Venerol 1999; 13(3): 228-9
2. Bergendorff O, Hansson C. Contact dermatitis to a rubber allergen with both dithiocarbamate and benzothiazole structure. Contact Dermatitis. 2007 May;56(5):278-80. doi: 10.1111/j.1600-0536.2007.01076.x.
3. Ceponis PJ, Cable R, Weaver LK. Don't Kick the Coral!, Wilderness & Environmental Medicine 2017.01.025, 28, 2, (153-155), (2017).
4. Koeppel M C, Bertrand S, Abitan R, Signoret R, Sayag J. Urticaria caused by cold. 104 cases. Ann Dermatol Venerol 1996; 123(10): 627-32
5. Kullavanijaya P, Sirimachan S, Bhuddhavudhikrai P. Mycobacterium marinum cutaneous infections acquired from occupations and hobbies. Int J Dermol 1993; 32(7): 504-7
6. Lacour J P, Elbaze P, Castenet J, Dubois D, Poudenx M, Ortonne J P. Diving suit dermatitis caused by Pseudomonas aeruginosa: 2 cases. J Am Acad Dermatol 1994; 31: 1055-56
7. Mathelier-Fusade P, Aissaoui M, Bakhos D, Chabane M H, Leynadier F. Clinical predictive factors of severity in cold urticaria. Arch Dermatol 1998; 134(1): 106-7
8. Okawa T, Hotta A, Sato, M, Takahashi S, Komori J, Aihara M. Allergic contact dermatitis caused by diethyl thiourea in a neoprene-containing wet suit. J Dermatol. 2018 Mar;45(3):365-366. doi: 10.1111/1346-8138.13873.
9. Qureshi H S, Dunne W M, Nakhleh R E. Unremitting ulcer in a Scuba Diver. Arch Pathol Lab Med 2001; 125: 450-2
10. Saltzer K R, Schutzer P J, Weinberg J M, Tangoren I A, Spiers E M. Diving suit dermatitis: a manifestation of Pseudomonas folliculitis. Cutis 1997; 59(5): 245-6
11. Weinberger LN, Seraly MP, Zirwas MJ. Palmar dermatitis due to a rubber escalator railing. Contact Dermatitis. 2006 Jan;54(1):59-60.
12. Sridhar J, Deo R. Marine and Other Aquatic Dermatoses. Indian J Dermatol. 2017 Jan-Feb;62(1):66-78. doi: 10.4103/0019-5154.198052. PMID: 28216728, PMCID: PMC5286756

# Diving Accidents 7

## DECOMPRESSION ILLNESS (DCI)

"The Bends", A "Hit"

"The only way to avoid decompression illness is either never to dive or never to ascend" (Unknown).

- The distinction between decompression sickness and arterial gas embolism is often impossible to distinguish by history or presentation and the two conditions may even occur concurrently so they have been clinically combined under the descriptive system umbrella of decompression illness (DCI) (Francis & Smith).
- Why some people suffer decompression illness whilst others who dive the same profile do not is often still a mystery. There is a huge variation in susceptibility to DCI between individuals and even within an individual from day to day. Certainly, many of the aggravating conditions and mechanisms of injury are still being elucidated.
- Pre-existing conditions, such as large patent foramen ovale (PFO) or other right-to-left intra-cardiac shunts and lung disease (IPAVA) have been shown to predispose to DCI.
- Rapid ascents or inadequate decompression stops are common in the dive profiles of divers who suffer DCI. One study showed they occurred in 50% of cases (Benton).
- Deep diving, repetitive diving, dehydration, alcohol intake, poor physical fitness, obesity, hypothermia, and increasing age have all been shown to increase the risk of DCI. Many divers get DCI for no apparent reason, so-called "unprovoked", their diving practice and profile being well within decompression limits. It is impossible to know whether it was a "random hit" or due to an individual DCI susceptibility. If they have a second episode of DCI then it is more likely that they are susceptible.
- The latency of the symptoms of neurological DCI may give an indication as to a predisposing factor. Immediate symptoms upon surfacing and within the first 5 minutes are more likely to be from arterial gas embolism, whilst symptoms occurring within the first 10-30 minutes may be associated with a large right-to-left intracardiac or intra-pulmonary shunting, such as intra-pulmonary arterio-venous anastomosis (IPAVA) or patent foramen ovale (PFO) (Wilmshurst & Moon).
- Even after a full recovery it is possible that the spinal cord and brain have sustained sub-clinical damage. A second episode of DCI could, and will, be clinically more serious due to loss of neuronal reserve.

Many recreational divers who suffer DCI are left with residual neurological deficits even after recompression therapy. Deficits can vary widely and have been noted to become more apparent months after the event.

Consider the risk that a second attack may be clinically more serious than the first (a possible, remote and major risk).

Consider the risk of the diver being susceptible to DCI and having another episode (a possible, rare and moderate risk).

Consider the risk of the diver having pulmonary pathology or a large PFO and having another episode (a proven, remote and moderate risk).

**A return to diving often depends on the motivation of the diver. Many divers, even after a single, fully-resolved DCI, will decide it is not worth the risk and stop diving. Another diver will want to continue diving even after an episode of DCI which has left a residual neurological deficit.**

**After a fully-resolved episode of DCI, we recommend no diving for at least four weeks.**

**If there have been cerebral, spinal, neurological, vestibulocochlear symptoms, or the presence of cutis marmorata, or if the symptoms far exceed the provocation, we suggest investigation with contrast bubble trans-thoracic echocardiography (after a delay of at least a month) to exclude a right to left shunt and/or high-resolution spiral CT lung scan to exclude overt lung pathology.**

**We reinforce the avoidance of aggravating factors and the limitation of depth and frequency of diving and the importance of a slow ascent (10 meters per minute or less) and increasing the length of decompression stops.**

**If there are residual neurological deficits or a second episode of DCI, we strongly recommend stopping any further diving activity. If the diver insists on continuing to dive, we suggest investigation as above and encourage them to wait as long as possible, avoid all aggravating factors and then limit diving to a maximum depth of 9 metres (30 ft), diving using Nitrox while still planning decompression on air tables and, ideally, no more than two dives a day (a single dive is always preferable and safer).**

## FACIAL BAROPARESIS

- This facial nerve palsy is thought to be a consequence of reduced axonal capillary blood flow in the setting of a defect in the bony covering of the tympanic segment of the facial nerve.
- Direct compression of the nerve can also occur due to the haemo-tympanum.
- A bony defect of the tegmen can also result in pneumocephalus and intracranial complications such as abscess and empyema.
- Compressive neuropraxia may occur during ascent from expanding trapped gas within the middle ear space. Air can also enter a normal facial nerve canal and cause compression by tracking along the chorda tympani nerve.
- It is only temporary but will tend to recur when the nerve palsy can become permanent.

Consider the risk of the palsy recurring and becoming permanent (a possible, remote and moderate risk)

**We would not recommend diving after an instance of facial nerve baroparesis.**

## PULMONARY BAROTRAUMA

Pneumothorax, Mediastinal and Cervical Emphysema

- Pulmonary barotrauma of ascent is caused by overdistension (not necessarily over-pressure) of the lungs. This will be due to either a sudden rapid ascent with inadequate air venting (a so-called "deserved" barotrauma) or due to localized air trapping within the lung tissue due to abnormal lung pathology or anatomy.
- The actual mechanism of lung rupture in the first instance is not known so it is impossible to predict the likelihood of recurrence should the person continue diving. If there is abnormal lung tissue which has caused barotrauma it would be very likely to happen again.

Consider the risk of another pulmonary barotrauma occurring, and the catastrophic consequences which can ensue.

**We do not recommend anyone with a history of pulmonary barotrauma to dive.**

**If a diver is determined to continue diving, they should first be fully investigated including an HRCT of the chest and assessed by a diving medical specialist (Goffinet).**

## INNER EAR BAROTRAUMA (IEBT)

- Inner ear barotrauma may involve haemorrhage into the cochlear duct, intra-labyrinthine Reissner or basilar membrane rupture or rupture of the round or oval window which sometimes persists as a peri-lymphatic fistula.
- Symptoms may include vertigo, tinnitus and hearing loss, but they are not dependable or reproducible. Tinnitus and high-frequency hearing loss are long-term complications.

Consider the risk of recurrence and acceleration of hearing loss and tinnitus (a plausible, remote and moderate risk).

**If the diver has made a full recovery from their IEB we would still strongly discourage diving. If the diver chooses to continue diving, it is important to reinforce careful ear equalization techniques, particularly the avoidance of forceful Valsalva manoeuvres.**

**A pure tone audiogram (PTA) should be recorded to have a baseline in case of developing future damage.**

## FURTHER READING:


1. Benton B J, Acute decompression illness (DCI): The significance of provocative dive profiles. Undersea Hyper Med 2001; 28(Supp): 25
2. Doolette D. Uncertainties in Predicting Decompression Illness. SPUMS J. 2000; 30 (1): 31-36
3. Francis TJR, Smith DJ, editors. Describing decompression illness. Kensington, MD: Undersea and Hyperbaric Medical Society, 1991.
4. Elliot D. Fitness to resume diving after decompression injury. SPUMS J 2001; 31(2): 90-2
5. Goffinet CMJ, Simpson G. Cerebral arterial gas embolism in a scuba diver with a primary lung bulla. Diving and Hyperbaric Medicine. 2019 June 30;49(2):141–144. doi: 10.28920/dhm49.2.141-144. PMID: 31177521.
6. Lindfors OH, Raisanen-Sokolowski AK, Hirvonen TP, Sinkkonen ST. Inner ear barotrauma and inner ear decompression sickness: a systematic review on differential diagnostics. Diving Hyperb Med. 2021 Dec 20;51(4):328-337. doi: 10.28920/dhm51.4.328-337. PMID: 34897597, PMCID: PMC8923696
7. Lippmann J, Lawrence C, Davis M. Scuba diving-related fatalities in New Zealand, 2007 to 2016. Diving Hyperb Med. 2021 Dec 20;51(4):345-354. doi: 10.28920/dhm51.4.345-354. PMID: 34897599, PMCID: PMC8920894
8. McQueen D, Kent G, Murrison A. Self-reported long-term effects of diving and decompression illness in recreational scuba divers. Br J Sports Med 1994; 28(2): 101-4
9. Moon R.E., Bove A.A. Transcatheter occlusion of patent foramen ovale: prevention of decompression illness? UHM 2004; 31(3): 271-274.
10. Ohm F, Leslie M. Round window membrane defects in divers. Laryngorhinootologie 1999; 78(4): 169-75
11. Parrell G J, Becker G D. Inner ear barotrauma in scuba divers. A long-term follow-up after continued diving. Arch Otolaryngol Head Neck Surg 1993; 119(4): 455-7
12. Rozycki SW, Brown MJ, Camacho M. Inner ear barotrauma in divers: an evidence-based tool for evaluation and treatment. Diving Hyperb Med. 2018 Sep 30;48(3):186-193. doi: 10.28920/dhm48.3.186-193. PMID: 30199891
13. Sheridan M F, Hetherington H H, Hull J J. Inner ear barotrauma from scuba diving. Ear Nose Throat Journal 1999; 78(3): 1186-7
14. Wilmshurst P, Bryson P. Relationship between the clinical features of neurological decompression illness and its causes. Clin Sci 2000; 99: 65-75

# Diving with Disabilities

# 8

## POINTS TO PONDER

Over the past years, there has been a transformation in the opportunity for people with disabilities to scuba dive. Organisations including Disabled Divers International (DDI), International Association for Handicapped Divers (IAHD) and Handicapped Scuba Association (HAS) have developed specific dive programs for disabled divers and specialised training courses for diving instructors and diving assistants to facilitate disabled divers to dive safely.

Traditional diving training organisations have added additional courses for disabled divers. The British Sub Aqua Club has a 'Diving for All' (DfA) program. PADI has an 'Adaptive Techniques Speciality Course'. Various dive centres and charter boats are improving accessibility for disabled divers to enter and exit the water.

Great ingenuity has been applied to adapt diving equipment for easier use. Even wheelchairs have been waterproofed, streamlined and powered for underwater transport. Full-face masks allow better communication.

Divers with quadruple amputation, autism, sight impairment, paraplegia, cerebral palsy, multiple sclerosis, and Down's Syndrome have all been trained to successfully dive in open water.

Divers with more severe disabilities have been able to dive in pools.

### Diving creates many therapeutic conditions:

- Weightlessness gives freedom to people with locomotion restrictions.
- Mobility, coordination, flexibility, and muscle tone are all improved.
- The hydrostatic pressure of water can aid in the reduction of oedema
- This freedom flows into an infusion of confidence, independence and sheer exhilaration (Naumann).

### Some general considerations include:

- The first rule to follow in considering potential problems is to ask the diver how they perceive it.
- The physical fitness and basic motor skills of people with disabilities are generally poorer than those of "able-bodied" peers but this is primarily due to a lack of opportunity to participate in physical activity programmes rather than physiological factors or motor development (Shephard).
- It is not appropriate to base a diver's potential ability simply on their supposed category as each diver will have unique abilities and qualities.

**The bottom line in diving is that the diver must be able to survive without injury to themselves or others. Many of the restrictions that impede the diver with disabilities are man-made and therefore can be man-overcome.**

## Adaptations include:

- Specifically designed diving courses.
- Specifically trained instructors and assistants
- Liberal time expectations.
- Equipment modifications.
- A team approach rather than buddy diving.
- Easy access to and from the water.

Many medical restrictions for diving safety are advised on the assumption that the diver is about to undertake an intense and condensed 'open water' dive course culminating in them diving in the open ocean in an independent buddy pair, after which they can dive unsupervised. This level of diving demands high levels of fitness, completion and demonstration of independent basic diving skills and the ability to save self and buddy in emergencies. Once this assumption is removed then lesser levels of fitness will incur less risk.

The main organisations which coordinate diving for disabled people have defined levels of diving competency by which divers with disabilities can be classified:

- Level A or 1 diver "has successfully met all standards, can take care of him or herself, help another diver in distress and perform a rescue. These divers are certified to dive with another buddy"
- Level B or 2 diver "has demonstrated the ability to handle emergencies, and in general, care for him or herself while scuba diving. This diver is unable to help another diver in distress. This diver should dive with two able-bodied certified dive buddies"
- Level C or 3 diver "has demonstrated the ability to safely dive with considerable assistance and could not be able to respond to an emergency, such as self-rescue. This diver must dive with two able-bodied certified dive buddies, one of whom must be trained in scuba rescue"

## For each disabled diver, several risks need to be considered:

Consider the risk of their disability reducing their ability to help themselves or others.

**Many risks may be reduced by modifying equipment, e.g., larger gauges, audible alarms, lighter regulators, low volume masks, full face masks, snorkels with purge valves, smaller tanks, larger buttons and levers, power inflators, full-length zips in wetsuits, webbed gloves, ankle weights, weight integrated buoyancy compensators, custom designed compass rigs, waterproof prostheses and propulsion units. Diving equipment design can be greatly improved for able-bodied divers by such considerations.**

**Many risks can be reduced by changing behaviour, e.g., interpreting written standards to specify the intention of a skill rather than the method of the skill. Educational videos can be closed-captioned. Instructors can learn the local sign language, e.g., Auslan in Australia, BSL in Britain, and ASL in the USA.**

Consider the risk of their disability predisposing them to dive-related problems.

The risk of decompression illness may be reduced by limiting the depth and frequency of diving and always incorporating a safety stop. Further precautions may include diving with enriched air but using air-based decompression tables.

Consider the risk of their disability mimicking decompression illness.

**This risk may be reduced if the baseline condition is well documented so any change can be monitored.**

Consider the risk of other conditions present.

Consider the risk of diving in very shallow water. Many of the early introductory dives are confined to 2 meters depth but this is the depth with the greatest rate of volume change with changing pressure. It is the depth where barotraumas (injuries caused by pressure changes) are most likely. Barotrauma to the middle ear and even pulmonary barotrauma has been documented as shallow as 1.2 meters.

**This book is not designed to cover the many disabilities which are relevant to diving. We mention some of the special considerations for common disabilities, which are commonly encountered.**

## AMPUTEES

Leg amputees, especially bilateral, may have trouble kitting up in rough conditions, finning and exiting the water. With good planning, all these can be easily overcome.

- Fins can be attached to stumps.
- Wetsuits can be custom-made to fit snugly over the stump.
- Stumps may have reduced sensation and are more prone to blisters and abrasions in wet conditions.
- Arm amputees may have difficulty kitting up, adjusting equipment, and exiting the water. Again, all these can be overcome with good planning.
- Prostheses can be made waterproof.

## BLINDNESS

### Severe sight impairment

- In Australia, this is defined as having less than 10% of sight, a visual field of 20°, or a corrected visual acuity of 6/60 or less.
- There is a need for two sighted buddies to act as guides, prevent collisions and help with rescues.
- A non-visual underwater communication system, either by touch or preferably audible using full face masks.
- Audible alarms may be useful for air content and ascent rates

## CEREBRAL PALSY

This is defined as "a disorder of movement and posture caused by a non-progressive brain disorder before the age of 2 years and often associated with birth trauma".

- The presence of complications such as epilepsy and intellectual disability is important.
- Spasticity and athetosis of the muscles may reduce coordination and locomotion. This mechanical inefficiency will cause early fatigue.
- Spasticity of the chest muscles could interrupt regular breathing. Spasticity, especially in the legs may be aggravated by cold.
- Because of damaged cerebral tissue, there is a possibility of an increased risk of decompression illness.

## DEAFNESS - TOTAL

- Defined as a hearing loss that renders it impossible to understand speech through hearing alone, even if a hearing aid is used. Hearing aids must be removed underwater and lip reading is not possible.
- Hearing plays little role whilst diving except for emergency diver recall procedures and hearing outboard motors when surfacing. Deaf divers communicating with sign language are at a distinct advantage when underwater.
- Deafness can sometimes be associated with middle ear pathology and with vestibular dysfunction.
- The middle ear must be able to equalise. If there is an anatomical deformity the structure should be confirmed with a CT scan.
- Training is helped by instructors skilled in sign language, videos with subtitles, adequate reading material, and classes, especially for deaf divers.

## INTELLECTUAL DISABILITY

- The cause of the disability may be relevant and should be determined and assessed. The presence of complications such as epilepsy, or hydrocephalus should be determined.
- The functional ability of the diver is most important. The severity may be graded into low, medium or high support needs.
- There is a reduced ability to think in abstract terms, in decision making and in poor short-term memory. These factors will reduce the awareness of danger and make close supervision compulsory.

## PARAPLEGIA

- The cause of the paraplegia needs to be determined and assessed, e.g., traumatic, spina bifida, or neurological decompression illness (DCI).
- Damaged neurological tissue, especially in the spine, may be more prone to DCI. This is especially relevant if the paraplegia was caused by a spinal decompression illness.
- Respiratory function may be restricted in lesions higher than T8 when intercostal muscles are weakened and diaphragmatic breathing will dominate. This can be aggravated by tight wetsuits.
- Such restriction will limit exercise tolerance but has no risk of pulmonary barotrauma since there is no air trapping.
- Diving can improve pulmonary vital capacity significantly in paraplegics (Novak).
- The lower body is unable to sweat so thermoregulatory control may be reduced. Shade is essential at the dive site, especially if in a hot climate (Gaisek).
- Bladder and bowel control programs may need to be adjusted. Paraplegics pool blood in their legs so when immersed they may have a significant immersion diuresis. Catheters can become kinked when fitting wetsuits.
- The condition of the skin, especially of the buttocks and the presence of pressure sores, needs careful attention to avoid infection with prolonged immersion.
- Legs trailing in the water, especially with loss of sensation, may be more prone to trauma and need measures to make them neutrally buoyant and have extra protection, e.g., knee and shin pads.
- The legs are susceptible to muscle spasms aggravated by cold. Some paraplegic divers use a Baclofen pump to reduce muscle spasticity. Generally, they have a 10-meter depth limit (Hacene).

# QUADRIPLEGIA

## Tetraplegia

- The same considerations that apply to paraplegics also apply to quadriplegics. However, the following additional points should also be considered.
- Thermoregulatory control is a bigger problem because of the greater reduction of available surface area for sweating. Staying in the shade, avoiding sitting in wetsuits, pouring cool water into wetsuits, spraying cool water onto the skin to promote evaporation and cooling, and ensuring an adequate fluid intake are all important cooling strategies.
- Divers with injuries at the T6 level and above will have damaged cardiac sympathetic innervation preventing reflex response to exercise. Maximum heart rates may be reduced to 110-130 per minute.
- Impairment of the respiratory muscles may lead to hypoventilation and make the diver more prone to carbon dioxide toxicity, especially as the density of the air increases with depth. This will also enhance nitrogen narcosis. Weakness of the respiratory muscles also decreases the ability to cough and clear secretions which predisposes to respiratory infections. Development of compensatory muscles in the neck may occur to reduce this risk.
- Reduced maximum heart rate, loss of use of respiratory muscles, and excessive pooling of blood in the lower body can cause light-headedness and dizziness with exercise.
- A potentially dangerous injury that can occur in people with a lesion above T6 is autonomic dysreflexia. The reaction can be triggered by an over-distended bladder or other painful stimulation resulting in high blood pressure, sweating, chills and headache.

# FURTHER READING:


1. Brown T. Physical Disability and Scuba Diving… in Medical Terms. The Undersea Journal, 1996 Second Quarter: 19-21
2. Gajsek U, Sieber A, Finderle Z. Thermal balance of spinal cord injured divers during cold water diving: A case-control study. Diving and Hyperbaric Medicine. 2020 September 30;50(3):256–263. doi: 10.28920/dhm50.3.256-263. PMID: 32957128.
3. Goodman S. Coaching Athletes with Disabilities: General Principles. 1993; Australian Sports Commission
4. Hacene B, Draulans N, Theys T. Problems with an intrathecal pump in a paraplegic scuba diver. Diving and Hyperbaric Medicine. 2018 June;48(2):110–111. doi. 10.28920/dhm48.2.110-111. PMID: 29888384.
5. Henrykowska G, Soin J, Siermontowski P. Scuba Diving as a Form of Rehabilitation for People with Physical Disabilities. Int J Environ Res Public Health. 2021 May 26;18(11):5678. doi: 10.3390/ijerph18115678. PMID: 34073170, PMCID: PMC8198635
6. Henrykowska G, Soin J, Pleskacz K, Siermontowski P. Influence of Scuba Diving on the Quality of Life of People with Physical Disabilities. Healthcare (Basel). 2022 Apr 20;10(5):761. doi: 10.3390/healthcare10050761. PMID: 35627898, PMCID: PMC9140659
7. Lin L Y. Scuba divers with disabilities challenge medical protocols and ethics. The Physician and Sports Med 1987; 15: 224-35
8. Meyers J. Adapting your instructional techniques within the PADI system. The Undersea Journal 1996 Second Quarter: 11-14

9. Morgan A, Sinclair H, Tan A, Thomas E, Castle R. Can scuba diving offer therapeutic benefit to military veterans experiencing physical and psychological injuries as a result of combat? A service evaluation of Deptherapy UK. Disabil Rehabil. 2019 Nov;41(23):2832-2840. doi: 10.1080/09638288.2018.1480667. Epub 2018 Jun 29. PMID: 29958006

10. Naumann K, Kernot J, Parfitt G, Gower B, Winsor A, Davison K. What are the effects of scuba diving-based interventions for clients with neurological disability, autism or intellectual disability? Diving Hyperb Med. 2021 Dec 20;51(4):355-360. doi: 10.28920/dhm51.4.355-360. PMCID: PMC8920902

11. Novak H F, Ladurner G. Significant increase of pulmonary vital capacity (VC) in scuba diving tetra- and paraplegics. Undersea Hyper Med 2000; 27(Supp): 46

12. Pedersen D M. Perceptions of high risk sports. Percept Mot Skills 1997; 85(2): 756-8

13. Shreeves J T. Accommodating – Not compromising: Teaching students with disabilities. The Undersea Journal, 1996 Second Quarter: 5-7

14. Shephard R J. Fitness in Special Populations. 1990; Chanpaign, Illinois; Human Kinetics Publishers Inc.

15. Stlefel V. Soaring Below. Alert Diver Mar/Apr 1996: 36-9

16. The International Association for Handicapped Divers Instructional Manual. Hjalmstauagen 8, S-186 36

17. Vallentuna, Sweden, 1997.

18. Walker K P. Diving with Care; training and medical aspects of diving with disabilities. Alert Diver Mar/Apr 1996: 40-1

# Drugs & Medications 9

## POINTS TO PONDER

- It is useful to ask the diver not only about any prescribed medication but also over-the-counter (OTC) medication and recreational drugs.
- The reason that a drug is taken needs to be determined and any associated risk with that condition assessed e.g. if a diver is taking a lipid-lowering drug, the possibility of ischaemic heart disease needs to be considered.
- What adverse drug reactions (ADR) may the drug have at atmospheric pressure, which may create risk in the underwater environment, e.g., sedation, vomiting, reduced exercise tolerance – e.g., beta-blockers may reduce the exercise tolerance of the diver, sedating antihistamines may cause drowsiness.
- Are there any interactions between drugs e.g., aspirin enhances the effects of sulphonylurea drugs.
- Will adverse drug reactions be enhanced by hyperbaric and diving conditions such as nitrogen narcosis, carbon dioxide toxicity, cold or fatigue e.g., sedating antihistamines may become even more sedating when combined with nitrogen narcosis?
- Will new adverse drug reactions occur because of hyperbaric conditions, e.g., bleomycin can cause pulmonary fibrosis when exposed to a high oxygen partial pressure.
- Will adverse drug reactions predispose the diver to any extra risk e.g., diuretics may cause dehydration which could predispose the diver to decompression illness.
- Will the delivery or absorption of the drug be affected by the diving or underwater environment e.g., drugs delivered by a transdermal patch may be more rapidly absorbed as the patch is more firmly applied to the skin underwater when any film of air beneath the patch is compressed. Seasickness can reduce the absorption of a drug prior to diving.

### For all the drugs listed:

Consider the risk of the condition for which the drug is being taken.

Consider the risk of each adverse drug reaction caused by the drug.

**This risk may be reduced if the diving doctor asks specifically for any adverse drug reactions common to the drug being taken and relevant to scuba diving. The following section may help. Moreover, whenever a new long-term drug is being commenced by a diver, a trial period of 3-4 weeks prior to diving should be observed to exclude immediate adverse drug reactions and drug idiosyncrasy.**

Consider the risk of any adverse drug reaction, which may be enhanced by diving. This risk may be reduced by limiting the depth of diving to avoid nitrogen narcosis.

Consider the risk of any condition that a drug could aggravate whilst diving.

Consider the risk of any change in the rate of absorption of the drug aggravated by diving.

**The adverse effects listed for each drug below do not cover all possible ADRs or possible risks. It is important to refer to the drug information to further assess ADR.**

## ALCOHOL

- One study showed that 57% of divers drank alcohol within 12 hours of diving. Older divers were generally heavier drinkers but younger divers were more likely to binge drink. 18% of divers had dived when considering themselves unfit to drive a car (St Leger-Douse).
- Young adult males are a high-risk group for drowning with alcohol shown to be a contributing factor (Mackie).
- Causes depression of the central nervous system reducing judgement, coordination and reaction time without the diver being aware of their impairment.
- Causes gastric irritation which could aggravate vomiting.
- Causes vasodilation of the skin accelerating heat loss and even leading to hypothermia and hypotension.
- Causes a diuresis which could aggravate dehydration and predispose to decompression illness.
- Binge drinking can induce cardiac dysrhythmias, especially atrial fibrillation (Ettinger).
- It may be a precipitating factor of exercise-induced anaphylaxis and asthma (Nichols).
- It may enhance the effects of nitrogen narcosis (Michalodimitrakis).
- Chronic alcohol abuse damages the heart, liver and brain.

**We advise anyone with a chronic alcohol abuse problem not to dive.**

Occasional drinkers should be advised not to take any alcohol 12 hours prior to diving and avoid excessive alcohol (more than four standard drinks) the night before diving. "Don't drink and dive".

## ANALGESICS

- The condition requiring analgesia should be determined and assessed. Anyone with acute pain or uncontrolled chronic pain for any reason should delay diving until the pain is controlled.
- Stronger analgesics containing codeine, dextro-propoxyphene or tramadol can have strong sedative side effects and could enhance the effects of nitrogen narcosis.
- Mild analgesics are relatively safe but due to the anticoagulant effects of aspirin, paracetamol seems preferable.
- Anyone with controlled chronic pain needs to consider the risk of the underlying condition.

**We do not recommend people requiring regular strong analgesics to dive.**

## ANTIBIOTICS

- The condition requiring the antibiotic needs to be determined and assessed.
- Many antibiotics cause nausea.
- Tetracyclines and quinolones may cause photosensitivity.

## ANTICOAGULANTS

Including coumarins such as warfarin, anti-platelet agents such as aspirin & clopidogrel, and direct thrombin inhibitors such as dabigatran and factor Xa inhibitors such as rivaroxaban and apixaban.

- Barotrauma is a common injury during diving, which often causes bleeding in the air- containing cavities of the body e.g., middle ear, sinus and lung.
- Neurological decompression illness may involve haemorrhage, especially in the spinal cord or inner ear.
- Minor skin trauma is common during diving.
- The condition for which the prospective diving candidate is on anti-coagulants needs to be taken into consideration e.g., atrial fibrillation, mechanical heart valve.

**We do not recommend anyone on anticoagulants to dive.**

## ANTI-CONVULSANTS

Including levetiracetam, gabapentin, lamotrigine, phenytoin, vigabatrin, carbamazepine, topiramate, pregabalin

- The condition requiring the anticonvulsant needs to be determined and assessed.
- Common adverse drug reactions include headache, sedation, dizziness, reduced concentration, ataxia, tremor and dysarthria. Some of the newer drugs may cause excitation and agitation.
- They may enhance the effects of nitrogen narcosis.

**We do not recommend anyone on anticonvulsants to dive.**

## ANTICHOLINERGICS

Including hyoscyamine, scopolamine, ipratropium

- The condition requiring the anticholinergic needs to be determined and assessed. It is usually used as an antispasmodic. Acute spasmodic pain may be suddenly disabling.
- Common adverse drug reactions include dry mouth, blurred vision and tachycardia.
- Causes a reduction in sweating which could affect thermo-regulation in hot climates.

## ANTI-DEPRESSANTS

Usually classified as:

- **Traditional** – amitriptyline, clomipramine, dosulepin, doxepin, imipramine, nortriptyline.
- **Selective serotonin reuptake inhibitors (SSRIs)** – citalopram, escitalopram, fluoxetine, fluvoxamine, paroxetine, sertraline
- **Serotonin and norepinephrine reuptake inhibitors (SNRIs)** – duloxetine, venlafaxine
- **Other** – trazodone, bupropion, mianserin, mirtazapine, moclobemide, agomelatine.
- **Monoamine oxidase inhibitors (MAOIs)** – phenelzine, tranylcypromine.
- Usually given for an affective mood disorder. The severity and stability of the illness need to be assessed.
- Tricyclic antidepressants can cause drowsiness, dizziness, dry mouth, fatigue, hypotension and delirium.
- RIMAs can cause nausea.

- MAOIs can cause postural hypotension and stimulant effects.
- SSRIs often cause nausea, especially when first taken. They can also cause agitation and sedation.
- Lithium can cause fine tremors, fatigue and nausea and diarrhoea. St John's wort can cause photosensitivity.
- An interaction between psychotropic medication and inert gas narcosis has been documented.
- All classes of anti-depressants entail a higher risk of convulsions; this is more common with bupropion and clomipramine.
- Anti-depressants potentially potentiate the anti-thrombotic effects of NSAIDs and warfarin, so they should be used in conjunction, due to the risk of bleeding worsening spinal DCS and/or ear/sinus barotrauma.

### We would only recommend diving if:

- On only one psychotropic medication, preferably a newer generation which is well tolerated than the traditional tricyclics, renowned for sleepiness and drowsiness.
- The diver is well-adjusted on the medication for at least 6 months, with no side effects and compliant with the medication.
- The condition for which the medication has been prescribed has been resolved and treatment is for maintenance only.
- Maximum depth of 15-20 metres to avoid interaction with inert gas narcosis.

**We would not recommend diving during the reduction of medication, if the underlying condition is not optimally controlled or if multiple psychotropic medications are required.**

## ANTI-EMETICS

### Hyoscine (Kwells, Scop patches)

- Commonly used by divers against seasickness, often in combination with antihistamines.
- Can cause drowsiness and, less commonly, impairment of memory and concentration, restlessness, dizziness, disorientation and confusion.
- Contamination of the finger from a patch can be transferred to the eye and cause pupillary dilation.

**Limited studies have suggested it is safe to use whilst diving.**

### Phenothiazines, e.g., prochlorperazine

- Not very effective for seasickness.
- Can commonly cause drowsiness and restlessness and rarely dystonic extrapyramidal reactions.

### Metoclopramide

- Not very effective for seasickness.
- Can cause drowsiness, restlessness, fatigue and lassitude. It rarely causes dystonic extrapyramidal reactions.

### Ondansetron

- Not very effective for seasickness.
- Side effects include headache, weakness, tiredness, chills, drowsiness and constipation.

## ANTIHISTAMINES

- Commonly used for allergic rhinitis, which is a common predisposing condition for middle ear and sinus barotrauma. Moreover, as they reduce and thicken secretions, they can cause a dry mouth and nasopharynx, which is also aggravated by breathing dry air. This may make equalisation of the middle ear more difficult.
- Commonly used as prophylaxis and treatment of seasickness. In space flight promethazine and meclizine are used for prophylaxis and intramuscular promethazine for treatment (Jennings).

### Sedating antihistamines, including promethazine, chlorphenamine, hydroxyzine, dimenhydrinate

- Commonly causes drowsiness, which seems to be enhanced underwater.
- Dimenhydrinate has been shown to affect different cognitive functions at 3 ATA (Taylor).

### Non-sedating antihistamines, including cetirizine, fexofenadine, loratadine, levocetirizine

- Being histamine H1 antagonists, they do not usually cause drowsiness and seem safer for allergic conditions.
- They are not very effective for seasickness.

**This risk may be reduced by taking the drug the evening before diving.**

**We do not recommend anyone on sedating antihistamines to dive.**

## ANTIHYPERTENSIVES

All drugs used for hypertension affect the autonomic nervous system. Side effects such as flushing, impotence, paraesthesia, and constipation may not all be relevant to diving but demonstrate the disruption of body function.

### Beta-blockers, including atenolol, bisoprolol, carvedilol, propranolol

- In moderate and high doses can cause bradycardia, and this chronotropic incompetence can limit heart rate modulation, and hence reduced cardiac response to exercise.
- Bronchospasm and allergic rhinitis can be exacerbated in atopic people, even years after the last attack, mediated through a decrease in FEV1 by bronchial beta-2 receptors.
- An anecdotal link between beta-blockade and immersion pulmonary oedema has been reported.
- Eye drops used for glaucoma can be absorbed systemically and rarely could cause adverse drug reactions as above. Systemic absorption can be reduced by gentle compression of the lacrimal punctate for two minutes after the instillation of the drops into the lower conjunctival sac.

### Calcium channel blockers including amlodipine, felodipine, nifedipine, verapamil

- Common adverse drug reactions include postural hypotension, drowsiness and weakness.
- A particular risk related to diving concerns the reversal of the central blood pooling effect of immersion upon exiting the water.

**Divers on calcium channel blockers should be advised to exit the water gradually whenever possible to allow blood pressure adaptation to occur.**

### ACE inhibitors, including captopril, perindopril, lisinopril, quinapril, enalapril Angiotensin II receptor antagonists, including candesartan, valsartan, telmisartan

- Common adverse drug reactions include persistent dry cough, hypotension, fatigue and dizziness.
- No diving-specific related risks are expected, widely considered to be the safest class of anti-hypertensives for blood pressure control in divers.

### Diuretics:

Thiazides including bendroflumethiazide, hydrochlorothiazide, indapamide Loop diuretics including frusemide, torsemide

- Adverse drug reactions include dizziness, muscle cramps and headaches.
- Electrolyte disturbances and dehydration can occur.

**We do not recommend anyone whose blood pressure control is not optimally controlled to dive (>160/100 mmHg), especially seeing the association between elevated blood pressure and immersion pulmonary oedema.**

We confirm that there is an appropriate cardiac response to exercise.

## ANTIMALARIALS

Commonly and importantly taken by divers whilst diving in the tropical waters of malarial areas.

- **Doxycycline** can cause nausea, vomiting, diarrhoea, allergy and photosensitisation. It can aggravate vaginal thrush infections and may reduce the efficacy of oral contraceptives. We would always emphasise the need for extra attention and precautions against sunburn.
- **Chloroquine** can cause headache, nausea and vomiting, diarrhoea, and rashes and may also cause photosensitivity
- **Proguanil** commonly causes heartburn (reduced by taking it after a meal with a glass of water and not lying down for 30 minutes), mouth ulcers (if occurs take folic acid tablets, 5 mg per day) and loose stools (self-limiting).
- **Atovaquone/Proguanil, (Malarone, Malanil)** is normally well tolerated but can cause headaches. Like proguanil alone, it can cause heartburn and mouth ulcers (see above).
- **Mefloquine** can commonly cause dizziness, disturbances of balance, depression, reduced sleep, "strange thoughts", vivid dreams, muscle aches and nausea. Less commonly it can cause spatial disorientation, interfere with fine motor coordination, visual disturbances, bradycardia and hallucinations. There has been concern that some of these symptoms could be confused for decompression illness after diving. It is not recommended for both divers and pilots.
- **Tafenoquine** One of the newer antimalarial drugs. The most common adverse events are headaches, back pain, dizziness, nausea, and diarrhoea. However, tafenoquine can cause severe haemolytic anaemia in people with G6PD deficiency and a quantitative G6PD test needs to exclude it before the drug can be prescribed.

**We do not recommend that anyone dives whilst taking mefloquine.**

## ANTIVIRALS

- Antiviral drugs are used to treat and prevent common infections e.g., herpes infection (both oral and genital), shingles and influenza A & B.
- Pre-exposure prophylaxis (PrEP), usually a combination of tenofovir and emtricitabine, is becoming widely accepted.
- Long-term antiviral drugs are used widely for HIV, chronic hepatitis B, hepatitis C and viral infections e.g., cytomegalovirus (CMV) in immunocompromised patients.

Some relevant adverse drug reactions of antivirals include:

Neuraminidase inhibitors, including oseltamivir, zanamivir, laninamavir, peramivir stomach cramps, bloating, chest pain or discomfort, diarrhoea, watery and severe, drooling, facial swelling, fast or irregular heartbeat.

### Interferon

- Malaise, fatigue, headache, depression, emotional lability, anxiety, rarely seizures.
- Nucleoside analogues including acyclovir, famciclovir, valaciclovir, zidovudine, remdesivir, ribavirin
- Generally, well tolerated but rash, itching, nausea, vomiting, diarrhoea, headache, light-headedness, and malaise.
- Nucleoside reverse transcriptase inhibitors (NRTIs) e.g., tenofovir, emtricitabine, zidovudine, didanosine, stavudine, lamivudine, abacavir
- Peripheral neuropathy, pancreatitis, stomatitis. Lactic acidosis with hepatic steatosis is a rare but potentially life-threatening toxicity.
- Non-nucleoside reverse transcriptase inhibitors (NNRTIs) e.g., efavirenz, delavirdine, nevirapine, rilpivirine
- Rash, hepatitis, dizziness, sleepiness, confusion, abnormal thinking, depersonalisation, impaired concentration, hallucinations.
- Protease Inhibitors (PIs), including saquinavir, ritonavir, indinavir, atazanavir
- Weakness, vomiting, dizziness, paraesthesia, hyperglycaemia and prolonged PR and QT intervals have all been reported.

## BRONCHODILATORS

Including aminophylline, salbutamol, salmeterol

- The use of bronchodilators usually reflects recent bronchospasm, which may carry specific risks related to asthma.
- Inhaled bronchodilators have a patchy effect within the lung so areas may be unaffected by the drug. It may lose some of its effects during a dive. Side effects include tremors in hands, dry mouth, headaches, palpitations, muscle cramps, nausea and vomiting, and diarrhoea.
- Aminophylline has been shown to relax the pulmonary arteriolar smooth muscle, reducing the efficiency of the pulmonary vascular filter bed which may allow venous nitrogen bubbles to enter the arterial circulation and predispose to arterial gas embolism.

## CAFFEINE

- High consumption can cause an increase in blood pressure and even induce cardiac dysrhythmias. It can also have a diuretic effect.
- It can protect against oxygen toxicity in rats (Bitterman).

## CANNABINOIDS

Cannabis, marijuana, dagga

- Cannabinoids have become legal in many parts of the world both for medical purposes and personal recreational use.
- The two main cannabinoids are delta-9-tetrahydrocannabinol (THC) and cannabidiol (CBD). THC is the chemical that is responsible for the psychoactive effects of cannabis including heightened senses, euphoria, sedation, impaired cognitive ability and hand-eye coordination, poor judgement, and lack of awareness, all of which are extremely hazardous to diver safety.

- Most medical CDBs do not contain THC and are not intoxicating, but there is little research about what other physiological effects CBDs would have on a diver's body. Commonly cited reasons for their use include chronic pain, multiple sclerosis, poorly controlled epilepsy and nausea and vomiting, especially from cytotoxics.
- Some CDB products are contaminated with THC (Lachenmeier).
- Random roadside saliva tests can detect THC for around twelve hours after use for people who use cannabis infrequently or 'recreationally'. However, for people who frequently use cannabis THC can be detectable for around 30 hours (Mather).
- Divers Alert Network (DAN) advise that 'divers stay out of the water for at least eight hours following smoking or ingestion of cannabis cookies or the oil to be confident there will be no psychoactive effects. This period should be extended if a large amount was ingested.' This focuses on the psychoactive effects of cannabis being 'the main acute safety concern during diving.'
- Whether the use of long-term non-intoxicating medical marijuana is hazardous to a diver's health is unknown. Possible side effects include dry mouth, diarrhoea, low blood pressure, light-headedness and drowsiness.

**We strongly recommend anyone addicted to THC and using it daily not dive.**

**We strongly advise any occasional user not to dive within 12 hours of smoking or ingesting THC.**

**We recommend anyone taking medical CBD use a pharmaceutical product that has been registered and has quality control of its ingredients (ensuring no contamination with THC).**

## COCAINE

"crack"

- Cocaine induces euphoria, a sustained mood elevation, increased energy and self-confidence, promotes talkativeness, alleviates fatigue and enhances mental alertness.
- Cocaine highs are usually intense but short-lived (15 to 90 minutes). It has a high potential for addiction and overdose.
- Cocaine is often cut with other substances. These sometimes include speed and fentanyl.
- Chronic cocaine use can lead to a range of cardiac complications. Acute myocardial infarction and myocardial ischaemia are the most common.
- It has been associated with sudden death syndrome in athletes even months after use.
- Regular intranasal use of cocaine may lead to damaging effects on the nasal mucosa. This ranges in severity from chronic rhinitis, reduced sense of smell, nosebleeds and septal perforation
- Smoking of crack cocaine can lead to a variety of acute pulmonary complications, including severe exacerbations of asthma and an acute lung injury syndrome associated with a broad spectrum of histopathologic changes ('crack lung')

**We do not recommend diving to anyone with a cocaine addiction.**

**We do not recommend diving to any occasional user within 12 hours of a 'high'.**

## CYTOTOXIC & IMMUNOSUPPRESSIVE DRUGS

Cytotoxic drugs including bleomycin, chlorambucil, carboplatin, cisplatin, cyclophosphamide, doxorubicin, gemcitabine, irinotecan, methotrexate, oncovin, procarbazine, paclitaxel

Immunosuppressive drugs, including adalimumab, infliximab, mycophenolate, rituximab, tacrolimus

- The reasons for taking the drugs must be determined and fully assessed e.g., malignant disease, multiple sclerosis, psoriasis, and rheumatoid arthritis.

- Cancer treatment has radically changed in the last twenty years with the introduction of immunotherapies which target the cancer cell. Nonetheless, chemotherapy is often combined with immunotherapy agents to enhance its effect.
- Chemotherapy will commonly cause severe nausea, vomiting, fatigue, general malaise, anaemia, malnutrition and dehydration.
- Cytotoxic drugs can cause pulmonary toxicity e.g., pneumonitis/fibrosis, cardiotoxicity, myelosuppression and immunosuppression. The latter can result in neutropenia and thrombocytopenia presenting as unexplained viral, fungal and bacterial infections, mouth ulcers, bruising and bleeding.
- Many cytotoxic drugs are cardiotoxic.
- Immunotherapy drugs are less toxic but still cause side effects e.g., flu-like symptoms, sinus congestion, and cough.

**We would not recommend anyone taking cytotoxics to dive. After cancer treatment has been ceased and a full recovery and convalescence completed diving should only be recommenced after a diving medical by a diving doctor to fully assess cardiac and pulmonary function.**

**Anyone on long-term immunotherapy treatment for non-cancer reasons should also have a diving medical to fully assess cardiac and pulmonary function.**

Certain cytotoxics are especially worthy of note:

## Bleomycin

- It is used in the treatment of testicular teratoma and can cause pulmonary toxicity in 3-10% of patients, usually in the form of pneumonitis/fibrosis (Simpson).
- Even in patients with no obvious pulmonary toxicity, the lungs were thought to be sensitised to raised levels of inspired oxygen, which can cause adult respiratory distress syndrome (ARDS) (Ayuso).
- For these reasons it was advised that anyone who had had bleomycin should avoid diving.
- However, a 2007 review of such patients who later had further surgery and were exposed to high levels of inspired oxygen during their anaesthetics showed no evidence of pulmonary complications (de Wit). Many such patients have since recommenced occupational diving with no complications. It was concluded that 'resumption of diving six to twelve months after an uncomplicated series of three or four cycles of BEP (bleomycin/etoposide/cisplatin) is completely acceptable. Caution should only remain for patients who develop clinical signs of pulmonary-function impairment during or shortly after bleomycin treatment.'

## Cisplatin

- Hyperbaric therapy seems to increase the cytotoxic effects of the drug in tissue impeding wound healing (Kindwall, Baud).

## Doxorubicin

- It is commonly used in the primary management of non-metastatic bladder carcinoma as well as lymphomas.
- Experimentally it was found to have 87% mortality in rats when combined with hyperbaric oxygen (HBO) exposure, presumably due to enhanced cardiac toxicity. There is no record of any diving-related incident but it is probably better avoided (Kindwall, Baude).

## DECONGESTANTS

Including pseudoephedrine, propylhexidine, naphazoline, oxymetazoline

- Probably the most common drug associated with diving. They are frequently used to aid middle ear equalisation and prevent sinus barotrauma in divers with mild upper respiratory congestion. They have been shown to be effective in reducing the incidence of middle ear barotrauma.
- Some divers who frequently have trouble equalising their ears take pseudoephedrine prophylactically.
- Pseudoephedrine can cause cardiac adverse drug reactions, including tachycardia, increased blood pressure, ventricular ectopic beats (VEs) and rarely atrial fibrillation.
- Pseudoephedrine is currently banned in sports by the World Anti-Doping Agency (WADA), as its stimulant activity is claimed to enhance performance.
- CNS stimulation includes palpitations, anxiety, vertigo, drowsiness, excitation, urinary retention and, rarely, hallucinations.
- As the effect of the drug wears off, there may be a rebound effect and the original congestion is actually worsened. Hence, the use of decongestants whilst diving may be associated with an increased incidence of aural and sinus barotrauma of ascent.
- Sympathomimetic stimulation may enhance nitrogen narcosis and reduce the convulsive threshold for oxygen toxicity, which is especially relevant if breathing enriched air (Thalmann).
- Pseudoephedrine has been shown not to affect psychometric performance at 3 ATA (Taylor).

**We do not recommend anyone taking pseudoephedrine to dive breathing enriched air.**

## DISULPHIRAM

This drug used to help alcoholics avoid alcohol blocks the production of superoxide dismutase (SOD) and could theoretically enhance the incidence of oxygen toxicity if exposed to multiple hyperbaric oxygen (HBO) treatments. There is no record of it adversely affecting anyone under HBO treatment or whilst diving.

## DIURETICS

Thiazides including bendroflumethiazide, hydrochlorothiazide, indapamide

Loop diuretics including frusemide, torsemide

- The reason for taking the diuretic must be determined and assessed, e.g., hypertension, congestive cardiac failure, recurrent leg swelling.
- Prolonged therapy can cause dehydration and electrolyte imbalance. Dehydration may predispose to decompression illness.
- When visiting hot climates, vasodilation and excessive sweating may enhance the effects.
- Other adverse drug reactions include weakness, fatigue, light-headedness and dizziness.

## HYPNOTICS

Sedative-hypnotics including nonbenzodiazepine receptor agonists (zaleplon, zolpidem, eszopiclone); short-acting benzodiazepine receptor agonists, (triazolam); intermediate-acting benzodiazepine receptor agonists (estazolam, temazepam); and selective melatonin agonists (ramelteon).

- The cause of insomnia needs to be determined and discussed. Emotional, psychiatric or addiction problems will need to be assessed.

- Many hypnotic drugs cause drowsiness well into the following morning. This effect may potentiate nitrogen narcosis.
- The short-acting benzodiazepines e.g., temazepam, and triazolam have an elimination half-life of 5-8 hours and are used by aircrews.

## HYPOGLYCAEMICS

The risks of diving with diabetes need to be assessed.

### Sulphonylureas, including glibenclamide, gliclazide, glipizide

- They potentiate glucose-stimulated insulin release from beta cells of pancreatic islets. Their most important adverse drug reaction is hypoglycaemia.
- They interact with several drugs to lower blood glucose, especially with aspirin, non-steroidal anti-inflammatory and sulphonamide drugs, but also with ACE inhibitors, beta-blockers, clofibrate and warfarin.

### Biguanides, including metformin

- They increase glucose uptake by skeletal muscle and adipocytes. Since they do not stimulate insulin release, they are less likely to cause hypoglycaemia unless combined with sulphonylurea.
- Lactic acidosis has been reported, usually when renal function is abnormal. Although rare, it can be fatal if not quickly corrected.

### Insulin

- Can cause hypoglycaemia with a sudden loss of consciousness.
- Insulin requirements may be increased by exercise and hyperbaric conditions.
- An autonomic neuropathy and the underwater environment may make the symptoms of hypoglycaemia less obvious.

### Thiazolidinediones, including pioglitazone, rosiglitazone

- They increase glucose uptake by skeletal muscle, liver and adipocytes. Since they do not stimulate insulin release, they are less likely to cause hypoglycaemia unless combined with sulphonylurea.

### Glinides, including repaglinide, nateglinide

- They promote insulin release by beta-islet pancreatic cells. Consequent to this, the main concern is the increased risk of hypoglycaemia occurring.

### DPP-4 inhibitors (gliptins), including vildagliptin, sitagliptin, saxagliptin, linagliptin, alogliptin

- They promote insulin release by beta islet pancreatic cells when required and decrease glucagon release when not required. They also modulate weight control by decreasing appetite. Their main side effects are gastrointestinal disturbance, flu-like symptoms and skin reactions; they have been associated with an increased risk of pancreatitis.

### SGLT2 inhibitors (flozins), including canagliflozin, dapagliflozin, empagliflozin

- They increase glucose excretion by blocking the renal sodium-glucose cotransporter 2. The main side effects are polyuria, increased risk of genito-urinary infections, osteopenia and electrolyte disturbances.

## LIPID-LOWERING DRUGS

Including atorvastatin, cerivastatin, gemfibrozil, simvastatin

- Taken for high serum lipids which are not controlled by diet alone.
- This is a risk factor for coronary artery disease which needs to be considered, especially if there are other risk factors present.
- Adverse drug reactions include myopathy with malaise, myalgia, fatigue, paraesthesia and neuropathy.

## NICOTINE

- Commonly applied as a dermal patch as an aid to stop smoking. Can cause vasoconstriction, elevated blood pressure and heart rate.
- The patch will be more closely applied to the skin during a dive and the absorption rate may be increased with a transitory exacerbation in side effects.

## NON-STEROIDAL ANTI-INFLAMMATORY DRUGS (NSAIDS)

Including indomethacin, diclofenac, naproxen, ibuprofen

- The reason for taking the NSAID must be determined and assessed.
- The commonest adverse drug reactions are heartburn, nausea and abdominal pain. Headache, dizziness, drowsiness and tinnitus can occur.
- Bronchospasm may be exacerbated in atopic people even years after their last attack. They must be taken with food, which may be difficult if seasick.
- They may potentiate other anti-coagulant medications.
- NSAIDs are being trialled as an adjunct to recompression therapy for decompression illness – one study shows efficacy with tenoxicam (Bennett).

## OPIOIDS

Including heroin, morphine, pethidine, fentanyl

- The reason for taking the narcotic needs to be determined and assessed.
- They may produce nausea, sedation, alterations in mood, reduced coordination, reaction time and judgement.
- Fentanyl may be delivered through a transdermal patch and absorption may be increased whilst diving, exacerbating side effects.

## ORAL CONTRACEPTIVE (OCP)

It has been suggested that oral contraceptive pill predisposes to decompression illness but there is no evidence to support it.

## PHOSPHODIESTERASE 5 (PDE5) INHIBITORS

Including sildenafil, tadalafil

- Phosphodiesterase-5 inhibitors were initially prescribed for male erectile dysfunction but have now been expanded for use in pulmonary hypertension and prostatic hyperplasia.

- PDE5 inhibitors are associated with dilation of the pulmonary vascular bed, with subsequent bypass of the pulmonary venous filter which usually traps circulating venous gas emboli post-diving.

**We do not recommend anyone on regular, daily PDE5 inhibitor therapy to dive.**

## PROTON PUMP INHIBITORS AND H2 BLOCKERS

The reason for taking the drug needs to be determined and assessed, e.g., active peptic ulcer disease, reflux oesophagitis.

- H2 receptor blockers, including cimetidine, ranitidine, famotidine

Generally, well tolerated but can cause headaches, tiredness, and drowsiness.

- Proton pump inhibitors, including omeprazole, lansoprazole, pantoprazole, esomeprazole, rabeprazole

Generally, well tolerated but can cause gastrointestinal upset, headache and dizziness and arthralgia.

## STEROIDS

Including prednisone, dexamethasone

- These are potent anti-inflammatory drugs. The reason for using the steroid needs to be determined and assessed.
- Prolonged steroid intake will cause many major side effects including hypertension, diabetes, osteoporosis, Cushing's syndrome, electrolyte disturbances and proximal myopathy.
- Steroids may enhance acute oxygen toxicity. This will not be of concern to the recreational diver unless they require hyperbaric treatment (Newman), Halpern).

## STEROID INHALERS

Including beclomethasone, budesonide, fluticasone

- Usually, prescribed for the treatment of allergic rhinitis, asthma and COPD.
- The use of the inhalers can cause oral and pharyngeal irritation and promote a monilial infection that could impede eustachian tube function.

## TRANQUILLISERS

Including alprazolam, chlordiazepoxide, diazepam, oxazepam

- The reason for taking the tranquiliser must be determined and assessed.
- Common adverse drug reactions include drowsiness, fatigue, muscle weakness and ataxia.
- Drowsiness may be enhanced by nitrogen narcosis.
- Many benzodiazepines have long half-lives e.g., diazepam has a half-life of about 80 hours.

**We would not recommend anyone taking benzodiazepines to dive.**

## VITAMINS

It has been suggested that Vitamin E and C, being anti-oxidants, could have a protective effect against oxygen toxicity (Bitterman, Money).

# FURTHER READING:


1. Ayuso L M, Martinez G, Souto M, Ortellis J. Intraoperative respiratory failure in a patient after treatment with bleomycin: previous and current intraoperative exposure to 50% oxygen. Eur J Anaesthesiol 1999; 16(1): 66-8

2. Bailly C, Thuru X, Quesnel B. Combined cytotoxic chemotherapy and immunotherapy of cancer: modern times. Cancer, 2020, Vol. 2, No. 1 1 doi: 10.1093/narcan/zcaa002

3. Baude J, Cooper JS. Hyperbaric Contraindicated Chemotherapeutic Agents. [Updated 2020 Aug 16]. In: StatPearls [Internet]. Treasure Island (FL): StatPearls Publishing; 2021 Jan-. Available from: https://www.ncbi.nlm.nih.gov/books/NBK560873/

4. Bitterman N, Schaal S. Caffeine Attenuates CNS Oxygen Toxicity in Rats. Brain Res 1995; 696: 250-3

5. Bitterman N, Eilander E, Melamed Y. Hyperbaric Oxygen and Scopolamine. Undersea Bio Res 1991; 18: 168-74 Bitterman N, Melamed Y, Ben-Amotz A. Beta-Carotene and CNS Oxygen Toxicity in Rats. J Appl Physiol 1994; 76(3): 1073-6

6. Bove A. Diving Medicine – Alcohol. Skin Diver 1987; 36(9): 32

7. Bove A. Diving Medicine – Cigarettes. Skin Diver 1987; 36(10): 22

8. Bove A. Diving Medicine – Cocaine. Skin Diver 1987; 36(11): 30

9. Bove A. Diving Medicine – Drugs and Diving. Skin Diver 1993; 42(6): 28-34

10. Brown M, Jones J, Krohmer J. Pseudoephedrine for the prevention of barotitis media: a controlled clinical trial in underwater divers. Ann Em Med 1992; 21(7): 849-52

11. Chesneau P, Thomas L, Mehdaoui H, Drault J N, Ketterle J. Does Cannabis play a role in scuba diving accidents? (letter) Presse Med 2000; 29(4): 188-9

12. Corey G R. Malaria and its preventative medication. Alert Diver Jan/Mar 2000: 31-2

13. Coupar-Smart J. Antidepressants and the diving medical (letter). SPUMS J 1995; 25(4): 216

14. Croft A M, Gardner P. Mefloquine for preventing malaria in on immune adult travellers. Cochrane Database Syst Rev 2000; 2: CD000138

15. Davis M. Scopoderm and Diver Performance. SPUMS J 1987; 17(1): 23-4

16. De Wit R, Sleijfer S, Kaye SB, Horwich A, Mead B, Sleijfer DT, Stoter G. Bleomycin and scuba diving: where is the harm? The Lancet. Volume 8, Issue 11, P954-955, November 01, 2007 DOI:https://doi.org/10.1016/S1470-2045(07)70321-2

17. Dive Magazine (Online) Legalisation of Cannabis Prompts Reconsideration of Diving Safety Advice http://divemagazine.co.uk/skills/8700-diving-cannabis-advice-dan

18. Dowse MS, Shaw S, Cridge C, Smerdon G. The use of drugs by UK recreational divers: illicit drugs. Diving Hyperb Med. 2011 Mar; 41(1):9-15

19. Fowler B, Adams J. Dissociation of the effects of alcohol and amphetamine on inert gas narcosis using reaction time and P300 latency. Aviat Space Environ Med 1993; 64(6): 493-9

20. Ettinger P O, Wan C F, De La Cruz C Jr, Weisse A B, Ahmed S S, Regan T J. Arrhythmias and the "Holiday Heart". Alcohol-associated cardiac rhythm disorders. Am Heart J 1978; 95: 555-62

21. Hoencamp E, van Dongen TT, van Ooij PJ, Wingelaar TT, Vervelde ML, Koch DA, van Hulst R, Hoencamp R. Systematic review on the effects of medications under hyperbaric conditions: consequences for the diver. Diving Hyperb Med. 2019 Jun 30;49(2):127-136. doi: 10.28920/dhm49.2.127-136. PMID: 31177519, PMCID: PMC6704002

22. Jennings R T. Managing space motion sickness. J Vestib Res 1998; 8(1): 67-70

23. Jones J S, Sheffield P W, White L J, Bloom M A. A double-blind comparison between oral pseudoephedrine and topical oxymetazoline in the prevention of barotrauma during air travel. Am J Emerg Med 1998; 16(3): 262-4

24. Josefsen R, Wester K. Cerebellar haemorrhage: a rare but serious complication in decompression disease. Tidsskr Nor Laegeforen 1999; 119(26): 3901-2

25. Halpern P, Teitelman U, Lauir A. Effects of methylprednisone on normobaric pulmonary oxygen toxicity in rats. Respiration 1985; 48(2): 153-8

26. Hamilton K, Laliberte M F, Heslegrave R. Subjective and Behavioural Effects Associated with Repeated Exposures to Narcosis. Aviat Space Environ Med 1992; 63: 865-9

27. Kindwall E P, Whelan H T. Hyperbaric Medicine Practice. 2nd edition 1999. Best Publishing Co., Flagstaff, A Z, USA.

28. Kroos B. Diving and Drugs. Imersed 1997; 2(4): 15-20

29. Lachenmeier DW, Habel S, Fischer B et al. Are side effects of cannabidiol (CBD) products caused by tetrahydrocannabinol (THC) contamination? F1000Research 2020, 8:1394

30. Levano B G. Taking drugs when you dive? Alert Diver 1999 Jan/Feb: 28-33

31. Lynch D A, Hirose N, Chernick R M, Doherty D E. Bleomycin induced lung disease in an animal model: correlation between computed tomography-determined abnormalities and lung function. Arad Radial 1997 Feb; 4(2): 102-7

32. Mackie I J. Patterns of drowning in Australia. 1992-97. Med J Austr 1999; 171(11/12): 586-9

33. Mamikoglu B, Corey J. Safety of antihistamine therapy. Curr Opin in Otolaryngology and Head and Neck Surgery 1998; 6; 75-79

34. Mather L. The issue of driving while a relevant drug, Δ9- tetrahydrocannabinol, was present in saliva: Evidence about the evidence. Griffith Journal of Law & Human Dignity. 2016;4(2):21-52.

35. Mekjavic I B, Passiad T, Sunberg C J, Eiken O. Perception of thermal comfort during narcosis. Undersea Hyperb Med 1994; 21(4): 9-19

36. Micchalodimitrakis E, Patsalis A. Nitrogen narcosis and alcohol consumption: a scuba diving fatality. J Forensic Sci 1987; 32: 1095-7

37. Miller B H. Sunning - And Still having Fun. Alert Diver Nov/Dec 1996: 37-9 Mims Annual 1999. 1 Chaddos Street, St Leonards NSW 2065, Australia.

38. Money F L, Strong P J. Underwater Diving, Oxygen Poisoning and Vitamin E (letter). NZ Med J 1972; 75: 34-5 Monteiro M G, Hernandez W, Figlie N B, Takahashi E, Korukian M. Comparison between subjective feelings to alcohol and nitrogen narcosis: a pilot study. Alcohol 1996; 13(1): 75-8

39. Murray J B. Psychophysiological aspects of motion sickness. Percept Mot Skills 1997; 85(3Pt2): 1163-7 Mutzbauer T S, Mueller P H, Tetzlaaff K, Sigg O, Neubauer B. Method for underwater application of nasal decongestants. Collection of manuscripts for the XXI Annual Scientific Meeting of the European Underwater and Baromedical Society (ed Gennser) 1998: 94-97

40. Newman J H, Falkerson W J, Kobayashi T, English D, Meyrick B, Brighan K L. Effects of methylprednisolone on lung oxygen toxicity in awake sheep. J Appl Physiol 1986; 60(4): 1386-92

41. Nichols A W. Exercise-induced anaphylaxis and urticaria. Clin Sports Med 1992; 11: 303-12 Nord D A. Over-the-Counter Drugs and Diving. Alert Diver May/June 1996: 39-42

42. O'Brien C P, Lyons F. Alcohol and the Athlete. Sports Med 2000; 29(5): 295-300

43. Perrine M W, Mundt J C, Weiner R I. When alcohol and water don't mix: diving under the influence. J Stud Alcohol 1994; 55(5): 517-24

44. Petersen E, Rome T, Ronn A, Bygbjey I, Larsen S O. Reported side effects to chloroquine plus proguanil, and mefloquine as chemoprophylaxis against malaria in Danish travellers. J Travel Med 2000; 7(2): 79-84

45. Querido AL. Diving and antidepressants. Diving Hyperb Med 2017 Dec;47(4):253-256. doi: 10.28920/dhm47.4.253-256. PMID: 29241236, PMCID: PMC6708605

46. Ralsey M J, Wardley-Smith B. Pressure Reversal of Narcosis Produced by Anaesthetics, Narcotics and Tranquillisers. Nature 1975; 257: 811-3

47. Rawlinson D. Antiviral agents for influenza, hepatitis C, herpesvirus, enterovirus and rhinovirus infections. Med J Aust 2001; 175(2): 122-6

48. Simpson A B, Paul J, Kaye S B. Fatal bleomycin pulmonary toxicity in the west of Scotland 1991-5: a review of patients with germ cell tumours. Br J Cancer 1998; 78(8): 1061-6

49. St Leger Dowse M, Bryson P, Gunby A, Fife W. Men and Women in Diving 1994. The Diving Diseases Research Centre, Fort Bovisand, Plymouth, Devon, UK.

50. St Leger Dowse M, Cridge C, Smerdon G. The use of drugs by UK recreational divers: prescribed and over the counter medications. Diving Hyperb Med 2011 Mar;41(1):16-21. PMID: 21560980

51. St Leger Dowse M, Cridge C, Shaw S and Smerdon G. Alcohol and UK recreational divers: consumption and attitudes. Diving and Hyperbaric Medicine. 2012;42(4):201-207.

52. Swenson E R, Hughes J M. Effects of acute to chronic acetazolamide on resting ventilation and ventilatory responses in man. J Appl Physiol 1993; 74(1): 230-7

53. Taylor D, O'Toole K, Auble T, Ryan C, Sherman D. The psychometric and cardiac effects of pseudoephedrine and antihistamines in the hyperbaric environment. SPUMS J 2001; 31(1): 50-7

54. Teicher B A, Holden S A, Cathcart K N. Effect of Various Oxygenation Conditions and Fluosol-DA on Cytotoxicity and Antitumour Activity of Bleomycin in Mice. J Natl Cancer Inst 1988; 80: 599-603

55. Thalmann E D. To mix or not to mix: is there conflict with pseudoephedrine and enriched air diving? Alert Diver Jan/Mar 2000: 8-10 Thomas J. Amphetamine and Chlordiazepoxide Effects on Behaviour Under Increased Pressure of Nitrogen. Pharm Biomed Behav 1973; 1: 421-26

56. Van Hulst RA, Rietbroek RC, Menno TWG, Schlosser NJJ. To dive or not to dive with bleomycin: a practical algorithm. Aviat Space Environ Med 2011 Aug;82(8):814-8. doi: 10.3357/asem.2816.2011. PMID: 21853861

57. Westerweel PE, Rienks R, Sakr A, Taher A. Diving with hypertension and antihypertensive drugs. Diving Hyperb Med 2020 Mar 31;50(1):49-53. doi: 10.28920/dhm50.1.49-53. PMID: 32187618 PMCID: PMC7276276

# 10

# Endocrine/ Metabolic Diseases

## POINTS TO PONDER

Endocrine diseases commonly have a hidden cause, an insidious onset and a very variable course. It is important to view their risk by considering:

- Is there an underlying cause which will create risk e.g., tuberculous or sarcoid destruction of the adrenal gland?
- What is the risk of the condition itself?
- What are the risks of complications?
- Simple changes in the diver's metabolic status can have significant implications in the diving environment, particularly the diver's hydration and conscious state.

## DEHYDRATION

- Dehydration from whatever cause is very significant because it is a risk factor for decompression illness (DCI).
- Common causes in divers include recent ethanol and caffeinated drink intake, seasickness, diarrhoea, excessive sweating when in tropical climates or with fever, jet travel (the air in aircraft is dry), high protein diets and diuretic use or abuse.
- During the dive, dehydration is exacerbated by breathing dry air and diuresis caused by both immersion and cold.
- Not only may dehydration predispose to DCI but the symptoms of dehydration can even mimic DCI, e.g., fatigue, and drowsiness.
- Dehydration will also reduce endurance performance and maximum oxygen utilization.

**All divers are recommended to aggressively avoid dehydration and ensure that their urine is a clear colour before diving (taking vitamin supplements may artificially colour urine).**

## DIABETES MELLITUS

Along with asthma, diabetes mellitus continues to be an ongoing debate in diving medicine. There are now many diabetics diving and several protocols have been formulated to enhance their safety.

| Selection and surveillance |
|---|
| Age >18 years |
| Delay diving until stable treatment established (6 months for oral hypoglycaemic agents and 12 months for insulin therapy) |
| No episodes of hypoglycaemia or hyperglycaemia requiring intervention or hospitalisation for at least 12 months |
| No episodes of hypoglycaemia unawareness |
| HbA1c <9% not more than one month before the initial and every annual assessment |
| No significant end-organ damage from diabetes mellitus, including renal, neurological, cardiac or ophthalmic complications |
| Diabetologist to carry out annual review in collaboration with diving medicine specialist, including evaluation for silent myocardial ischaemia with exercise electrocardiography testing and functional exercise testing. |
| Candidate documents intent to follow the established and agreed protocol to permit safe diving, understand the interplay between diving and blood glucose control, demonstrates optimal knowledge of the use of a blood glucose measuring device and aware that they need to seek advice if any change in clinical status occurs. |

| Scope of diving |
|---|
| Diving should be limited to ideally one single dive per day (if 2 dives entertained, a surface interval of well over 2 hours should be undertaken), and should be planned to avoid: |
| • Depths deeper than 30 msw (100 fsw) |
| • Durations > 60 minutes total dive time |
| • Obligatory decompression stops |
| • Overhead environments (wreck or cave penetration) |
| • Situations that provoke hypoglycaemia (long arduous dives or cold exposure) |
| Diving buddy/dive leader should be informed of diver's diabetic status and is trained with the appropriate response in the eventuality of an emergency situation |
| Diving buddy should not be diabetic themselves |

- Diabetes is characterized by hyperglycaemia and deranged metabolism. They may present acutely with dehydration, ketoacidosis and hyperventilation or chronically with lethargy and general ill health.
- Diabetics may be at risk of decompression illness (DCI) due to their hyperosmolarity, dehydration, increase in blood viscosity and increased thrombotic tendency.
- The main risk to the treated diabetic is the problem of hypoglycaemia, and its occurrence and repercussions underwater. It is more likely to occur with insulin but can also occur with certain classes of oral hypoglycaemic agents.
- The symptoms of hypoglycaemia include confusion, sweating, tachycardia, altered consciousness and convulsions. The warning symptoms may be perceived differently or confused in the underwater environment, especially under the influence of nitrogen narcosis.
- Long-standing insulin-dependent diabetics can even have a phenomenon known as "hypoglycaemia unawareness" thought to be due to hypothalamic desensitization to falling serum glucose (Braatvedt).
- Hypoglycaemia may be aggravated by incidental infections.
- Hypoglycaemia may be aggravated whilst diving because of the variable conditions which can affect even the most well-planned dive. A planned quiet dive may result in prolonged maximal exertion due to unexpected currents, cold temperatures or rescue efforts.

- Hypoglycaemia may be aggravated by the hyperbaric conditions themselves which may increase the rate of glucose metabolism (O'Malley) although it is thought to be the partial pressure of oxygen and not the ambient pressure that is responsible (Elanayake).
- Hypoglycaemic symptoms may also be confused with symptoms of decompression illness. The other concern with diabetes is the risk of long-term complications, especially the premature onset of coronary artery disease, hypertension, peripheral vascular disease and autonomic neuropathy (which may hide ischaemic cardiac pain). Symptoms of neuropathy such as paraesthesia, numbness and mononeuritis may be confused with symptoms of DCI.
- If the diabetic deliberately creates hyperglycaemia to protect against hypoglycaemia, then they may run the risk of provoking ketoacidosis with acidosis stimulating hyperventilation. On top of this, they may be at a higher risk of DCI as described above.
- In the past few years, the equipment for testing and recording blood sugar levels has become smaller, simpler and more accurate and better suited for use in the diving environment.

Consider the risk of hyperglycaemia causing ketoacidosis resulting in hyperventilation (a possible, remote and moderate risk).

Consider the risk of hypoglycaemia causing reduced consciousness and even convulsions (a proven, regular and major risk).

**This risk can be minimised by following a strict protocol as tabled below.**

| Glucose management on the day of diving |
|---|
| Blood glucose > 9 mmol/L (162 mg/dL), stable or rising, on 3 blood glucose measurements 60 minutes, 30 minutes and immediately prior to diving |
| Delay dive if blood glucose < 9 mmol/L (162 mg/dL) or > 16.7 mmol/L (300 mg/dL) |
| Rescue medications should be available, including oral glucose sources on the diver themselves, as well as parenteral glucagon at the dive-site |
| If hypoglycaemia is noticed underwater, the diver should do a controlled ascent with the buddy, establish positive buoyancy, ingest oral glucose and leave the water safely |
| Check blood glucose post-dive, including up to 12-15 hours post dive due to late decrements in blood glucose |
| Ensure adequate hydration on days of diving |
| Log all details of dives, including blood glucose levels and changes in medication/status |

Consider the effect of diabetic complications on diving, particularly ischemic heart disease but also neuropathy (a proven, regular and moderate risk).

**These risks may be reduced by being physically fit and performing regular exercise. If over 45 years old a stress ECG and stress echocardiogram is recommended (Jendle).**

**We would not recommend any diabetic patient with end-organ damage, multiple therapies or poorly controlled glycaemic control to dive.**

We would only recommend a diver with diabetes mellitus to dive if all the criteria set above are met and are reviewed annually with no deterioration in clinical status, with the diver being well aware of the criteria and his compliance with the protocols in place prior, during and after planned dives.

# HYPOTHERMIA

We include this section for information so that the relevance of hypothermia to divers can be reinforced.

- Rapid immersion in cold water can cause cardiac dysrhythmias resulting in sudden death or uncontrolled hyperventilation. Even a small increase in minute volume can be perceived as a restricted air supply and may induce panic, especially in the inexperienced (Doubt).
- Water conducts heat 25 times faster than air so the body will cool much more rapidly underwater. Heat is especially lost from the head, groin and axillae. The scalp is especially important as the vessels do not vasoconstrict with cooling.
- Hypothermia is defined as a body core temperature of 35°C or less but even lesser amounts of cold stress can cause physiological problems. Thermal comfort does not necessarily relate to thermal status.
- Symptoms of hypothermia include reduced capabilities to make judgements resulting in irrational behaviour and reduced muscle strength, speed and coordination.
- Cold causes vasoconstriction of peripheral blood vessels, reducing skin and muscle blood flow which results in an expansion of the central blood volume leading to diuresis. Upon rewarming the diver is significantly dehydrated, a risk factor for decompression illness (DCI).
- Being warm at the beginning of a dive may cause the diver to have an increased nitrogen uptake compared to later in the dive when they get cold and the hypothermia retards off-gassing and predisposes them to DCI.
- Divers specifically at risk of hypothermia include children and those with a thin physique.

# JET LAG

- Many divers fly to distant dive sites and dive immediately after they arrive. Jet lag is common if you cross more than 3 time zones.
- Symptoms include fatigue, difficulty concentrating, loss of appetite, irritability and disorientation.
- As a rough guide, symptoms will last TZ/2 days after a flight to the west and TZ/1.5 after one to the east, where TZ is the number of time zones crossed.
- Whilst flying it is advised to avoid alcohol and caffeine, drinks plenty of fluids, take brief strolls and adjust your watch to the destination time at the beginning of the flight and adjust meals and sleep patterns to this time.
- After arrival adjust your habits to the new time. Avoid naps. Short-acting hypnotics may be helpful the first night or two.

**We recommend that divers do not dive the first day after a flight that crosses 4 time zones or more and that they are particularly careful to avoid dehydration.**

# THYROID DISEASE

Hyperthyroidism, Grave's Disease, Hypothyroidism, Thyroiditis

- Many of the symptoms of thyroid disease are disabling and can be confused with decompression illness (DCI). It may take many months or years of treatment to achieve a stable well-controlled thyroid state.
- Hyperthyroidism can cause tachycardia and more serious dysrhythmias, heart failure, proximal myopathy and muscular weakness. Even if treated with anti-hyperthyroid drugs 50% will relapse. Radioactive iodine treatment will often result in a hypothyroid state which needs thyroid hormone supplement.
- Hypothyroidism can be very insidious in its onset with general malaise, lethargy, motor retardation, bradycardia and heart failure. Thyroid hormone levels and normal physiology return very slowly even when treatment is commenced.

Consider the risks of the symptoms causing disability whilst diving.

**We would not recommend diving until the diver had stable, normal thyroid hormone levels and is free of symptoms of over or under function. Usually, they need to improve physical fitness after such as illness before diving is commenced.**

## FURTHER READING:


1. Adolfsson P, Ornhagen H, Jendle J. The benefits of continuous glucose monitoring and a glucose monitoring schedule in individuals with type 1 diabetes during recreational diving. J Diabetes Sci Technol 2008 Sep;2(5):778-84. doi: 10.1177/193229680800200505. PMID: 19885260, PMCID: PMC2769802

2. Adolfsson P, Ornhagen H, Jendle J. Accuracy and reliability of continuous glucose monitoring in individuals with type 1 diabetes during recreational diving. Diabetes Technol Ther 2009 Aug;11(8):493-7. doi: 10.1089/dia.2009.0017. PMID: 19698062

3. Bantin J. So you think you can take the cold? Diver 1999; 44(1): 36-38

4. Bonomo M, Cairoli R, Verde G, Morelli L, Moreo A, Delle Grottaglie M, Brambilla MC, Meneghini E, Aghemo P, Corigliano G, Marroni A. Safety of recreational scuba diving in type 1 diabetic patients: the Deep Monitoring programme. Diabetes Metab 2009 Apr;35(2):101-7. doi: 10.1016/j.diabet.2008.08.007. Epub 2009 Feb 28. PMID: 19251448

5. Bove A A. Diabetics and diving. SPUMS J 1995; 26(2); 106-7

6. Braatvedt G. Hypoglycaemia in adult patients with diabetes mellitus. New Ethicals 2000; April: 53-60

7. Davies D. SPUMS statement on diabetes. SPUMS J 1992; 22: 31-32

8. De L Dear G, Pollock N, Uguccioni D, Dovenbarger J, Feinglos M N, Moon RE. Plasma glucose responses in recreational divers with insulin-requiring diabetes. Undersea Hyperb Med Fall 2004;31(3):291-301. PMID: 15568417.

9. Doubt T J. Physiology of exercise in the cold. Sports Med 1991; 11: 367-81

10. Edge CJ, St Leger Dowse M, Bryson P. Scuba diving with diabetes mellitus--the UK experience 1991-2001, Undersea Hyperb Med Jan-Feb 2005;32(1):27-37. PMID: 15796312

11. Edmonds C, A Diabetic Damsel in Distress. SPUMS J 1996; 26 (4): 223-5

12. Ekanayake L, Doolette D J. Effects of hyperbaric oxygen treatments on blood sugar levels and insulin levels in diabetics. SPUMS J 2001; 31(1): 16-20

13. Francis J. Immersion Hypothermia. SPUMS J 1998; 28(3): 25-29

14. Miller I. Cold and the diver. SPUMS J 1990; 20(1): 33-9

15. Gherardin T. Jet Lag. A problem for "long haul" travellers. Aust Fam Physician 1999; 28(8): 833

16. Jendle J, Adolfsson P, Ornhagen H. Swedish recommendations on recreational diving and diabetes mellitus. Diving Hyperb Med 2012 Dec;42(4):231-3. PMID: 23258460

17. Jendle J, Adolfsson P, Pollock N. Recreational diving in persons with type 1 and type 2 diabetes: Advancing capabilities and recommendations. Diving Hyperb Med 2020 Jun 30;50(2):135-143. doi: 10.28920/dhm50.2.135-143. PMID: ∫ PMCID: PMC7481121

18. Jendle J, Adolfsson P. Continuous Glucose Monitoring Diving and Diabetes: An Update of the Swedish Recommendations.

J Diabetes Sci Technol 2020 Jan;14(1):170-173. doi: 10.1177/1932296819826584. PMID: 30712367, PMCID: PMC7189164

19. Johnson R. Insulin-dependent diabetes mellitus and recreational scuba diving in Australia. Diving Hyperb Med 2016 Sep;46(3):181-185. PMID: 27723022

20. Johnson R. A day in the life of a diabetic diver: the Undersea and Hyperbaric Medical Society/Divers Alert Network protocol for diving with diabetes in action. Diving Hyperb Med. 2016;46(3):181-185.

21. Koufakis T, Karras S N, Mustafa O G, Karangelis D, Zebekakis P, Kotsa K. Into the deep blue sea: A review of the safety of recreational diving in people with diabetes mellitus. Eur J Sport Sci 2020 Feb;20(1):1-16. doi: 10.1080/17461391.2019.1606286. Epub 2019 Apr 23. PMID: 31013208

22. Kruger D F, Owen S K, Whitehouse F W. Scuba diving and diabetes (letter). Diabetes Care 1995; 18(7): 1074

23. Lerch M, Lutrop C, Thurm U. Diabetes and diving: can the risk of hypoglycaemia be banned? SPUMS J 1995; 26(2): 62-6

24. Lormeau B, Pichat S, Dufaitre L, Chamouine A, Gataa M, Rastami J, Coll-Lormeau C, Goury G, Francois A-L, Etien V, Blanchard J-L, Herve D, Sola-Gazagnes A. Impact of a sports project centered on scuba diving for adolescents with type 1 diabetes mellitus: New guidelines for adolescent recreational diving, a modification of the French regulations. Arch Pediatr 2019 Apr;26(3):161-167. doi: 10.1016/j.arcped.2018.12.006. Epub 2019 Mar 15. PMID: 30885605 DOI: 10.1016/j.arcped.2018.12.006

25. Manfredini R, Manffredini F, Fersini C, Conconi F. Circadian rhythms, athletic performance and jet lag. Br J Sports Med 1998; 32(2): 101-6

26. O'Malley E, Berkowicz L, Suttle K, Cetina S, Fife C. Blood glucose in diabetics undergoing hyperbaric oxygen therapy. UHMS Gulf Chapter, Annual Scientific Meeting, 1998, March 12-15, Galverston, Texas

27. Pieri M, Cialoni D, Marroni A. Continuous real-time monitoring and recording of glycemia during scuba diving: pilot study. Undersea Hyperb Med May-Jun 2016;43(3):265-72. PMID: 27416695

28. Pollock NW, Uguccioni DM, Dear GdeL. Diabetes and recreational diving: guidelines for the future. Diving Hyperb Med. 2006: 36;29-34.

29. Seldon W L. You're getting verrry sleepy – combating jet lag on long-distance dive trips. Dive Training 1999; 3(9): 82-85

30. Taylor L, Mitchell S. Diabetes as a contraindication to diving: Should old dogma give way to new evidence? SPUMS J 2001; 31(1): 44-48

31. Uguccioni D, Dovenbarger J. The Diabetes Question. Alert Diver Jan/Feb 1996: 21-3

32. YMCA Protocol for Diabetes 1995.

33. Uguccioni D, Pollock M, Moon R. Blood glucose response to single and repetitive dives in insulin-requiring diabetics: a preliminary report. Undersea Hyper Med 1998; 25 (Suppl): 52

34. Williamson J. Some diabetics are fit to dive but which ones? SPUMS J 1995; 26(2): 70-72

# 11

# Ear, Nose and Throat Diseases

## POINTS TO PONDER

### EAR

- The middle ear is the only air-containing organ which needs active pressure equalization whilst diving. The inability to equalize the middle ear causing barotrauma is by far the most common injury experienced by divers (Monnot, St Leger Dowse). For details on equalizing the middle ear, see Appendix A.
- On the descent, a pressure differential of only 60 mmHg between the middle ear and water in the external canal may cause symptoms. The tympanic membrane is inwardly stretched causing pain, oedema and haemorrhage. The mucosa within the middle ear cavity becomes congested and can exude a transudate or haemorrhage depending on the severity and rapidity of the barotrauma. This will cause a feeling of ear blockage and a reduction in hearing. Because it reduces the volume of the middle cavity, it may initially relieve the pain.
- When the pressure differential reaches 90 mmHg, the eustachian tube (ET) may lock up preventing equalization regardless of the method and necessitating ascent to reduce the pressure and unlock the tube.
- A pressure differential between 100 and 500 mmHg, may result in perforation of the tympanic membrane. This may cause instant relief of symptoms but, if cold water enters the middle ear cavity, it may also cause vertigo and nausea.
- On the ascent, the middle ear will usually vent air passively when the pressure differential with the nasopharynx is about 15 mmHg.
- Even during the course of a dive, equalization of the middle ear can become more difficult due to the drying of the nasopharynx whilst breathing dry air.
- Repetitive multi-day diving leads to a significant decrease in compliance and an increase in peak pressure (overpressure) in the middle ear (Meyer).
- The tympanic membrane is about ten times bigger than the oval window. The ossicles give a leverage advantage of 1.7 to 1. The sudden violent movement of the tympanic membrane can therefore lead to a pressure wave within the inner ear that can be transmitted to the round window causing its rupture or damage to the membranes within the inner ear.
- Pressure transmitted from the chest to the CSF (via the neck vessels) during a forceful Valsalva manoeuvre can also be transmitted to the inner ear via the cochlear aqueduct. This usually occurs at a time when there is relative negative pressure in the middle ear and these changes combined can result in an outward rupture of the round window.
- Vertigo and vomiting, common symptoms of inner ear pathology, are extremely dangerous if experienced underwater. Vertigo can lead to total disorientation and loss of connection with the surface. Vomiting can cause gagging and retching and cause the free flow of air through the regulator. Both may lead to panic.

- Hearing is not an essential sense when diving and communication with hand signals is a distinct advantage. Poor hearing per se is not a problem in sports diving.
- During their careers, naval and occupational divers do not show a greater loss in hearing than non-diving personnel indicating that with correct training and supervision diving per se does not cause permanent hearing loss. There is some evidence that this occurs in sports diving too (Sames, Wingelaas, Haussmann, Taylor).

## SINUSES

- The sinus ostia are normally patent and communicate with the nasal cavity and nasopharynx and allow passive equalization with both descent and ascent.
- Sinus barotrauma is usually self-limiting and rarely dangerous, usually causing severe facial pain or toothache, headache and blood in the mask, which will usually stop further diving and make the rest of the day miserable. There may be a sudden "pop" during depth changes thought to be due to haemorrhage stripping off the mucosa from the sinus wall.
- Serious complications can occasionally occur including orbital hematoma, facial subcutaneous emphysema, pneumocephalus with air in the subdural space and sinusitis with its possible complications, e.g., brain abscess and empyema.
- Sinus barotrauma occurs on both descent (about 66 %) and ascent (about 33 %).
- Repeated sinus barotrauma may cause scarring of the sinus ostia or ducts and predispose to further barotrauma and chronic sinusitis.

## UPPER RESPIRATORY TRACT

Allergic Rhinitis

Hayfever

- This commonly causes nasal mucosal swelling, a profuse clear watery nasal discharge and sneezing. It will predispose to aural and sinus barotrauma.
- It commonly occurs in atopic individuals who might also suffer from asthma.
- A common treatment is a daily oral antihistamine.
- Consider the risk of middle ear and sinus barotrauma (a proven, regular and minor risk).
- Consider the risk of the diver taking sedating antihistamines causing drowsiness underwater (a plausible, regular and moderate risk).

**This risk may be reduced by using non-sedating antihistamines. Diving should be avoided whilst suffering from any symptoms.**

### Bifid Uvula

- This should alert one to the possibility of a submucosal cleft palate. It can be associated with hypoplasia of the eustachian tubes (ET) and occurs in 2-3% of the population.

Consider the risk of poor ET function predisposing to middle ear barotrauma (a possible, remote and minor risk).

**This risk may be reduced by ensuring there is good ET function with Valsalva manoeuvres and reinforcing the methods of equalization. See Appendix A.**

## Cleft Palate

- It is nearly always associated with poor Eustachian tube (ET) function, even if a full repair of the defect has successfully occurred.
- The teeth can be crowded and deformed interfering with easy retention of the regulator's mouthpiece.

Consider the risk of poor ET function predisposing to middle ear barotrauma (a possible, remote and minor risk).

**This risk may be reduced by ensuring there is a good ET function with a Valsalva manoeuvre and reinforcing the methods of equalization. See Appendix A.**

Consider the risk of difficulty holding the regulator's mouthpiece in the mouth.

**This risk may be reduced by a soft silicone mouthpiece or even a custom-made mouthpiece. Most people with significant cleft palates will not have adequate ET function for diving.**

## Laryngectomy

- The normal reason for such surgery is a malignancy of the neck. It results in loss of sensation and protective reflexes to the airway. If a total laryngectomy has been performed a tracheostomy is required.

Consider the risk of inhalation of water into the trachea (a plausible, regular and major risk).

Consider the risk of malignancy causing easy fatigue and malaise.

**It is not feasible to dive with a tracheostomy and we would not recommend anyone to dive after a partial laryngectomy.**

## Laryngocele

- This is an air-filled dilation of the larynx near the vocal cords and is uncommonly seen in musicians playing large brass instruments.
- The swelling will enlarge with a Valsalva manoeuvre but usually having a wide neck will easily deflate.

Consider the risk of the swelling enlarging on the ascent causing an upperairway obstruction (a possible, rare and major risk).

**We would recommend an ENT assessment to ensure the laryngocele is wide-necked so there is no danger of air trapping.**

## Nasal Polyps

- Usually associated with chronic infection, nasal obstruction orallergic rhinitis.
- Even after treatment, they have a high recurrence rate.

Consider the risk of middle ear and sinus barotrauma (a plausible, regular and minor risk).

**The risk may be reduced by prior treatment of the cause of the polyps, treatment of the polyps themselves, ensuring normal eustachian tube function before diving and reinforcing techniques of middle ear equalization. See Appendix A.**

## Nasal Septal Deviation

- Seen commonly even in people with no history of nasal trauma. In severe cases, the deviation interferes with nasal breathing and predisposes to sinus barotrauma.

- There is some evidence to show that eustachian tube (ET) function may also be diminished.

Consider the risks of sinus barotrauma (a plausible, remote and minor risk).

**This risk may be reduced by informing the diver of the problem and advising that any dive be aborted if symptoms occur. If symptoms recur, surgical correction of the deviation may be advisable.**

Consider the risk of aural barotrauma (a possible, remote and minor risk).

**This risk may be reduced by ensuring there is a good ET function with a Valsalva manoeuvre and reinforcing the methods of equalization. See Appendix A.**

## Sinusitis

- Sinusitis will predispose to sinus barotrauma (see points to ponder).
- In a recent survey of 921 divers, 49% admitted to having suffered sinus barotrauma during their diving career (Lindfors).
- Recurrent sinus infections may be aggravated by allergic sinusitis, irritation by cigarette smoke, snorting cocaine, overuse of decongestant sprays, fumes or mechanical obstruction.
- Common anatomical abnormalities include obstructed infundibulum, conchal bullosa and sinus cysts and polyps. Functional endoscopic sinus surgery (FESS) has been shown to be very effective in correcting these abnormalities and allowing divers to return to diving (Granstrom).
- Even after endoscopic surgery serious complications can occur. These may be aggravated by repeated forceful Valsalva manoeuvres (Parell).
- Chronic sinusitis should first be controlled by medical management.

Consider the risks of sinus barotrauma (a plausible, regular and minor risk).

**This risk may be reduced by delaying diving until all infections and swelling are resolved. Any underlying cause should be identified and treated. If a mechanical obstruction is suspected a CT scan is recommended as soon as possible after symptoms develop. If a mechanical abnormality is found, endoscopic surgery may help.**

**We do not recommend diving to anyone with any active sinus infection or blockage.**

We tell anyone who has had recurrent sinusitis of the known serious risks and that it is impossible to predict if they will occur.

We advise them to avoid forceful Valsalva manoeuvres and to descend cautiously. If they experience sinus pain, they should abort their dive. If they have recurrent sinus barotrauma, they should seek specialist treatment.

**It is common that when a diver has limited time to recover before a diving commitment, or the condition occurs whilst on a diving expedition, they will try and reduce the nasal congestion by taking pseudoephedrine or nasal decongestant drops. This practice may work but, if the effect of the drug wears off before the end of the dive, there may be a rebound effect with an increase in the risks.**

## Tracheostomy

- Bypassing the larynx leaves the airway with no protective reflexes or sphincter.

Consider the risk of aspiration of water directly into the trachea and bronchial tree (a plausible, regular and major risk).

**We would not recommend diving for anyone with a tracheostomy.**

## Upper Respiratory Infection

Including Tonsillitis, Pharyngitis, Laryngitis

- The mucosal swelling and increased mucus production of the nasopharynx predispose to sinus and aural barotrauma with a spread of the infection.

Consider the risks of sinus and aural barotrauma (a proven, regular and mild risk).

**These risks may be reduced by treating the condition and waiting until all symptoms have subsided.**

# EXTERNAL EARS

## Ear Plugs

- Ear plugs will create an air space in the outer ear between the plug and the tympanic membrane that will lead to a reverse middle ear barotrauma of descent, (also known as a "reverse ear" or "external ear squeeze").
- This can also be caused by a tight diving hood.
- There are fenestrated earplugs designed for surfers to keep the wind out of their ears. These may be safe for diving but there is no reason to use them underwater.

Consider the risk of "reverse ear" (a plausible, regular and minor risk).

**We recommend that no earplugs ever be used whilst diving.**

## Facial Jewellery

- Prominent or dangling rings can become entangled with the mask strap or diving hood and cause lacerations to the skin.
- Fish can be attracted by bright jewellery and pull on them quite forcibly with their mouths.
- Nose studs can be pushed into the nose by a mask being knocked off and push the inner rod into the nasal septum.
- Tight hoods can push ear studs into the skin over the mastoid area.

## Earwax

- Ear wax is formed in the outer third of the external canal. It is produced continuously and provides waterproofing of the skin of the outer ear.
- If it is pushed inwards by washing, swimming, fingertips or cotton buds it will tend to accumulate high in the external canal and form plugs of ear wax that can cause impaction with an ear-plug effect and a risk of reverse middle ear barotrauma.
- A build-up of ear wax will also cause retention of skin debris and water in the outer ear predisposing to otitis externa.

**We recommend excessive accumulation of ear wax is removed by the use of wax softening drops, and, if necessary, gentle ear syringing or suction under medical supervision. Do not syringe if there is a history of tympanic membrane perforation or middle ear surgery.**

## Exostoses

- Bony outgrowths in divers commonly occur bilaterally on the walls of the external ear canal, commonly in response to long exposures to cold water (Ito).
- The narrowed canal is more prone to blockage with cerumen, debris and dead skin and will easily retain moisture predisposing to recurrent otitis externa and otorrhea.

- If the canal is completely blocked an asymmetrical caloric stimulus with vertigo can occur with submersion.

Consider the risk of recurrent otitis external (a proven, regular and minor risk).

Consider the risk of sudden vertigo on submersion (a proven, rare and moderate risk).

**We recommend surgical removal (canaloplasty) if there is associated hearing loss, external canal occlusion or recurrent otitis externa.**

### Otitis Externa

- Some people are prone to recurrent infection, especially if they have narrow canals, large exostosis or eczema of the outer auditory canal.
- Diving will predispose to infection and prevent any concurrent infection from resolving.
- The infection can be excruciatingly painful, with Pseudomonas aeruginosa being the commonest pathogen.

Consider the risk that acute otitis externa will be aggravated by diving (a proven, regular and minor risk).

**This risk may be reduced by immediate treatment and waiting until the pain has settled before resuming diving. If diving with otitis externa, ensure the canal is clear of debris and is well-dried after diving. The ear should be dried by putting a clean tissue at the opening of the external canal. Do not dry with a cotton bud. Warm air from a hair drier may also be used.**

## TYMPANIC MEMBRANE AND MIDDLE EAR

### Cholesteatoma

- The presence of a squamous epithelial sac within the middle ear cleft causes disruption to the architecture of the middle ear and surrounding tissues, and usually causes a chronic discharge and often a peripheral perforation of the tympanic membrane.
- It may form granulation tissue and polyps within the middle ear cavity.
- As the cholesteatoma expands it erodes surrounding bone so the middle ear cavity may communicate with the semi-circular canal or the cranial cavity. Any middle ear barotrauma, especially of ascent, could cause air or infection to also extend and even form an abscess.
- It is difficult to treat and may become chronic.
- Treatment involves surgical removal of diseased tissue and reconstruction of the middle ear and ossicular chain.
- Reduced hearing is inevitable.

Consider the risks of middle ear barotrauma causing air and infection to extend into the semi-circular canals or cranial cavity (a plausible, regular and major risk).

**We would not recommend anyone with a cholesteatoma to dive.**

### Effusion

- The presence of a serous effusion in the middle ear usually reflects poor eustachian tube (ET) function.
- This may be due to an ongoing underlying pathology e.g., nasopharyngeal infection, allergy, nasal obstruction or recent barotrauma from diving or flying.

Consider the risk of middle ear barotrauma (a proven, regular and mild to moderate risk).

**This risk may be reduced by determining and treating the cause of the effusion and allowing it to be completely reabsorbed with normal ET function before diving is resumed.**

**We would not recommend anyone with a middle ear effusion to dive.**

## Grommets

Tube myringotomy

- These small aerating tubes are usually inserted through the tympanic membrane because of the inadequate eustachian tube (ET) function.
- This may be due to an ongoing underlying pathology, e.g., nasopharyngeal infection, allergy or nasal obstruction.
- Common types of grommets are naturally extruded from the tympanic membrane (TM) usually after six to twelve months, sometimes before the reason for their insertion has resolved.
- Tympanosclerosis may form on the tympanic membrane as a result of middle ear dysfunction.

Consider the risk of water entering the middle ear and causing vertigo and infection (a proven, regular and moderate risk).

**We would not recommend anyone with grommets in their tympanic membranes to dive.**

We advise anyone with a history of grommets to wait three months after their extrusion before diving, to have their doctor check full healing of the TM, that ET function is normal and stress the importance of equalizing the ear regularly on the descent and not waiting for any sensation of pressure.

## Mastoidectomy – simple

- The removal of the cortex of the mastoid and opening of all the cells and antrum is usually performed for acute mastoiditis, which does not settle with antibiotics alone.
- Although the mastoid antrum is drained, the middle ear and external auditory meatus remain intact.

Consider the risk that the original infection also damaged the tympanic membrane, leaving it scarred and less mobile, predisposing to middle ear barotrauma (a possible, remote and moderate risk).

**The risk may be reduced by checking that the operative site is fully healed, the tympanic membrane is mobile and that the Eustachian tube function is normal.**

We would recommend diving if healing is complete and the tympanic membrane is mobile with normal ET function.

## Mastoidectomy – radical/modified

- Excision of the mastoid cells or mastoid process (often in association with tympanoplasty) is usually performed for cholesteatoma and occasionally for chronic infection.
- The external ear often becomes combined with the mastoid space to form a large cavity that allows cold water to circulate and produce a significant caloric effect on the labyrinth to aggravate vertigo. This can occur not just on entering the water but when passing through thermoclines.
- It is usually accompanied by severe hearing loss.

Consider the risk of causing vertigo when the outer ear floods with cold water, whilst diving (a plausible, regular and moderate risk).

**We would not recommend diving after such a procedure.**

## Monomeric tympanic membrane

- This can be seen as a "blowout" or "ballooning" from the tympanic membrane during a Valsalva manoeuvre.
- It may be caused by part of the tympanic membrane healing, often after a perforation, by lack of the formation of the middle fibrous layer.
- Usually, the diver is completely unaware of the abnormality.
- Because of its thinness and distensibility, it may perforate before any warning symptoms are apparent.

Consider the risk of an increased incidence of perforation of the tympanic membrane (a plausible, remote and moderate risk).

**The risk may be reduced if the diver is made aware of the abnormality and advised on the importance of equalizing the ear regularly on the descent and not waiting for any sensation of pressure.**

## Myringoplasty
## Tympanoplasty

- Surgical restoration of a perforated tympanic membrane (TM) by grafting.
- The fact that the perforation did not heal spontaneously may reflect an ongoing pathology.

Consider the risk of scarring and adhesions from the graft reducing the mobility and elasticity of the TM and making it more liable to re-perforate (a plausible, regular and moderate risk).

Consider the risk of any underlying pathology in the middle ear.

**This risk may be reduced if the TM is mobile and not retracted.**

**If the TM is mobile with normal eustachian tube function, we will recommend diving.**

## Ossicular Prostheses

Total Ossicular Replacement Prostheses (TORP)

Partial Ossicular Replacement Prostheses (PORP)

- Reconstruction of the integrity of the middle ear and ossicular chain is usually performed because of cholesteatoma or chronic middle ear infection.
- The main purpose of the procedure is to improve hearing.
- Complications of the procedure include prosthesis extrusion and slippage, penetration of the TORP through the stapes footplate into the vestibulum (Pau).

Consider the risk of middle ear barotrauma causing damage to the ossicular chain and oval window leading to severe hearing loss (a possible, rare and major risk).

**This risk may be reduced by ensuring early and adequate middle ear equalization when diving.**

**We would not recommend anyone to dive after this procedure.**

## Perforation of the Tympanic Membrane

Ruptured eardrum

- The perforation may indicate the presence of an ongoing pathology in the middle ear.

- The perforation will allow water to enter the middle ear from the external ear, possibly causing sudden vertigo and leading on to infection.

Consider the risk of water entering the middle ear and causing vertigo and infection (a proven, regular and moderate risk).

**This risk may be reduced by having any underlying pathology treated and allowing the perforation to heal or be repaired by myringoplasty prior to diving.**

**We would not recommend anyone with a patent perforation to dive. We normally advise divers to allow at least six weeks for an acute perforation to heal and strengthen and to have a diving doctor assess the tympanic membrane and eustachian tube function before diving.**

## SCARRING OF THE TYMPANIC MEMBRANE (TM)

- Previous injury or infection can cause atrophic changes and retraction of the tympanic membrane.
- The pressure differential across the TM required to cause a rupture has been shown to be significantly lower in the presence of an atrophic scar. The resultant perforation was also typically larger (Jensen).

Consider the risk of the TM being easily ruptured whilst diving causing vertigo, infection and a chronic perforation (a plausible, remote and moderate risk).

**This risk may be reduced by careful attention to middle ear equalization.**

**If the TM is retracted and/or severely scarred we would strongly discourage diving.**

### Stapedectomy

- The removal and replacement of the stapes with a prosthesis are usually performed for otosclerosis.
- Forced or explosive middle ear equalization could subject the oval window to excessive movement with the danger of dislodgment of the prosthesis and damage to the membrane and inner ear.
- A survey of ENT specialists regarding their recommended restrictions and clinical experiences failed to demonstrate a consensus (Harrill).

Consider the risk of dislodgment of the plate of the stapes with damage to the membrane and inner ear (a plausible, rare and major risk).

**This risk can be reduced by careful attention to ear equalization and avoidance of any forced Valsalva manoeuvres.**

**We would not recommend anyone to dive after this procedure.**

### Tympanosclerosis

- White plaques are sometimes seen in the tympanic membrane, which represents tympanosclerotic changes within the fibrotic layers.
- They may occur as a result of recurrent or chronic otitis media or secondary to trauma such as myringotomy or grommet insertion.
- Large tympanosclerotic plaques can occur in the anterosuperior portion of the TM and fix the manubrium of the malleus. They may also form around the ossicles and result in their fixation.

Consider the risk that the TM is less elastic and more prone to perforation (a plausible, remote and moderate risk).

**This risk may be reduced by ensuring the TM is fully mobile when the middle ear is equalized and reinforcing the**

**middle ear equalizing techniques.**

**In most cases, tympanosclerosis is an incidental finding and very mild.**

**If it is severe and associated with deafness or reduced eustachian tube function, a specialist assessment should be obtained.**

## INNER EAR

Labyrinthitis, Vestibular neuritis

- These conditions of the inner ear can cause sudden, recurrent attacks of vertigo, nausea and vomiting.
- They are usually caused by viral infections and are self-limiting within a few weeks.
- However, the inner ear may be permanently damaged by the infection and chronic dizziness, fatigue, and disorientation, as well as tinnitus and hearing loss can ensue.

Consider the risk of sudden incapacitation underwater from an attack of vertigo (a plausible, remote and moderate risk).

**We would not recommend diving to anyone suffering from this condition.**

### Meniere's Disease

Labyrinthus hydrops

- There is dilation of the endolymphatic system of the inner ear with denervation of the sensory components of the cochlea and vestibular apparatus. No cause is known.
- Acute symptoms occur suddenly and include vertigo, nausea and vomiting. Attacks may last from 20 minutes to 24 hours.
- Attacks occur randomly and may not occur for extended periods.
- It causes progressive deafness and tinnitus.
- Even after surgery, inner ear dysfunction may continue.

Consider the risk of sudden incapacitation underwater from an attack of vertigo (a plausible, remote and moderate risk).

Consider the risk of barotrauma to the middle or inner ear aggravating the hearing loss (a plausible, remote and moderate risk).

**We would not recommend diving to anyone with this history.**

## POSITIONAL VERTIGO

Benign Paroxysmal Positional Vertigo (BPPV), Post-traumatic

- Considered to be due to free-floating particles called canaliths (calcium carbonate crystals) in the semi-circular canals. It is sometimes seen in patients with a history of recent head injury.
- Symptoms include sudden attacks of vertigo, nausea and rarely vomiting which can be provoked by head movement.
- Diagnosed using the Dix Hallpike manoeuvre.
- It is usually self-limiting but can be recurring.
- It can be treated with canalith repositioning manoeuvres (Epley).

Consider the risk of sudden incapacitation from an attack of vertigo (a plausible, regular and moderate risk).

**We would not recommend diving to anyone with this active condition. The recommencement of diving should be decided after a specialist assessment.**

## Deafness – partial

- Hearing plays little part whilst diving underwater. In fact, anyone fluent in sign language is at a distinct advantage. However, anyone with unilateral deafness is totally dependent on one good ear and they are therefore far more vulnerable to permanent disability if the healthy ear is damaged.
- The commonest injury sustained whilst diving (apart from abrasions) is aural barotrauma. The commonest serious complication of aural barotrauma is hearing loss.
- The deafness may be caused by pathology within the middle or inner ear and therefore increases the risk of local barotrauma.

Consider the risk of an abnormality of the middle or inner ear predisposing to barotrauma. Even if someone is totally deaf, this can still cause significant morbidity with pain and haemorrhage (a proven, regular and moderate risk).

**The risk may be reduced by determining the exact nature of the deafness and ensuring there is normal Eustachian tube function.**

Consider the risk of additional hearing loss occurring and greatly worsening their disability (a proven, rare and major risk).

**The risk may be reduced by educating the diver about the potential risks, emphasizing the importance of early middle ear equalization on the descent and ensuring their technique is effective.**

It is crucial to have an accurate assessment of the cause of deafness. If there are no other risks associated with deafness and there is normal ET function, we leave the choice to the diver, after ensuring the diver understands the high incidence of middle ear barotrauma and the possibility of inner ear barotrauma.

## Tinnitus

- Buzzing in the ears is a common symptom in the older diver due to presbyacusis.
- Common causes are exposure to noise e.g., gunfire, loud music, head injury, Meniere's disease, aminoglycosides and trauma.
- In its severest form, it can be distracting and disabling.
- The commonest diving injury is barotrauma of the ear, which can cause a permanent exacerbation of pre-existing tinnitus.

Consider the risk of the condition causing tinnitus (if known).

Consider the risk of sustaining an aural barotrauma to the ear, which can cause a permanent exacerbation of pre-existing tinnitus.

**The risk may be reduced by early and adequate middle ear equalization.**

**We inform the diver of the risks, and in the absence of other pathology, we let them decide.**

## Temporomandibular joint (TMJ) dysfunction

- Diving regulator mouthpieces are typically made of silicone rubber and held in place by a bite platform, with the mandible positioned anteriorly to properly position the regulator, thus leading to uneven loading of the TMJ joint.
- Symptoms of diving-related temporomandibular dysfunction (TMJD) include pain and fatigue in the TMJ and muscles of

mastication (e.g., masseter or temporalis), TMJ crepitus and clicking, headache and tinnitus.

- Risk factors include female gender, inexperience with diving, bruxism, clenching, biting on the mouthpiece and poor-quality mouthpieces.
- Excessive occlusal pressure on a mouthpiece can also cause non-barotraumatic tooth fracture (odontocrexis).
- Exacerbation of pre-existing TMJD is likely, with referred otalgia being common and should not be mistaken for aural barotrauma.

**Custom mouthpieces are recommended for divers with TMD to optimize underwater occlusal forces.**

## FURTHER READING:


1. Alzamil K S, Linthicum F H Jr. Tympanosclerosis. Am J Otol 1999; 20(5): 686-7
2. Butler F K, Bove A A. Infraorbital hypesthesia after maxillary sinus barotrauma. Undersea Hyperbaric Med 1999; 26(4): 257-9
3. Bellini M J. Blindness in a diver following sinus barotrauma. J Laryngol Otol 1987; 101: 386-89
4. Brown M, Jones J, Krohmer J. Pseudoephedrine for the prevention of barotitis media: a controlled clinical trial in underwater divers. Ann Em Med 1992; 21(7): 849-52
5. Edmonds C. Sinus barotrauma. A bigger Picture. SPUMS J 1994; 24(1): 13-19
6. Elliott EJ, Smart DR. The assessment and management of inner ear barotrauma in divers and recommendations for returning to diving. Diving Hyperb Med 2014 Dec;44(4):208-22. PMID: 25596834
7. Fagan P, McKenzie B, Edmonds C. Sinus barotrauma in divers. Ann Oto Rhinol Laryngol 1976; 85: 61-4 Goldman R W. Pneumocephalus as a consequence of barotrauma. JAMA 1986; 255: 569-72
8. Granstrom G, Ebenfelt A, Ehrenstrom L, Nilsson A, Westin T, Ornhagen H. Management of recurrent sinus barotrauma in divers with functional sinus surgery (FESS). Proceedings of the 12th International Congress on Hyperbaric Medicine, International Joint Meeting. Oriani G, Wattel F, eds. 1996: 97-105
9. Haider T, Stanek G. Otitis Externa in tropical diving and swimming. Wien Klin Wochenschr 1992; 104(2): 39-41
10. Harrill W C, Jenkins H A, Coker N J. Barotrauma after Stapes Surgery: A Survey of Recommended Restrictions and Clinical Experiences. Am J Otol 1996; 17(6): 835-46
11. Hausmann D, Laabling S, Hoth S, Plinkert PK, Klingmann C. Assessment of the peripheral hearing system of sport divers. Undersea Hyperb Med Nov-Dec 2011;38(6):515-26
12. Hermans P E, Bracke P G, Demeyer IV. Pneumocephalus due to barotrauma: CT demonstration (letter). AJR Am J Roentgenol 1992; 159(6): 1351-2
13. Hollis L, Bottrill I. Menieres Disease. Hosp Med 1999; 60(8): 574-7
14. Ito M, Ikeda M. Does cold water truly promote diver's ear. Undersea Hyperb Med 1998; 25(1): 59-62
15. Jensen J H, Bonding P. Experimental pressure induced rupture of the tympanic membrane in man. Acta Otolaryngol Stockh 1993; 113(1): 62-7
16. Kieser J. Sinus barotrauma presenting as acute dental pain (letter). S Afr Med J 1997; 87(2): 184
17. Kozuka M, Nakashima T, Fukuta S, Yanagita N. Inner ear disorders due to pressure change. Clin Otolaryngol 1997; 33(2): 106-10
18. Lechner M, Sutton L, Fishman JM, Kaylie DM, Moon RE, Masterson L, Klingmann C, Birchall MA, Lund VJ, Rubin JS. Otorhinolaryngology and Diving-Part 1: Otorhinolaryngological Hazards Related to Compressed Gas Scuba Diving: A Review. JAMA Otolaryngol Head Neck Surg 2018 Mar 1;144(3):252-258. doi:10.1001/jamaoto.2017.2617.

19. Lechner M, Sutton L, Fishman JM, Kaylie DM, Moon RE, Masterson L, Klingmann C, Birchall MA, Lund VJ, Rubin JS. Otorhinolaryngology and Diving-Part 2: Otorhinolaryngological Fitness for Compressed Gas Scuba Diving: A Review. JAMA Otolaryngol Head Neck Surg 2018 Mar 1;144(3):259-263. doi: 10.1001/jamaoto.2017.2616. PMID: 29450499

20. Lindfors OH, Raisanen-Sokolowski AK, Suvilehto J, Sinkkonen ST. Middle ear barotrauma in diving. Diving Hyperb Med. 2021 Mar 31;51(1):44-52. doi: 10.28920/dhm51.1.44-52. PMID: 33761540, PMCID: PMC8313771

21. Lindfors OH, Räisänen-Sokolowski AK, Suvilehto J, Sinkkonen ST. Sinus barotrauma in diving. Diving Hyperb Med. 2021 Jun 30;51(2):182-189. doi: 10.28920/dhm51.2.182-189. PMID: 34157734; PMCID: PMC8426117.

22. Livingstone DM, Lange B. Rhinologic and oral-maxillofacial complications from scuba diving: a systematic review with recommendations. Diving Hyperb Med 2018 Jun 30;48(2):79-83. doi: 10.28920/dhm48.2.79-83.PMID: 2988837, PMCID: PMC6156823

23. Livingstone DM, Smith KA, Lange B. Scuba diving and otology: a systematic review with recommendations on diagnosis, treatment and post-operative care Diving Hyperb Med 2017 Jun;47(2):97-109. doi: 10.28920/dhm47.2.97-109. PMID: 28641322 PMCID: PMC6147252

24. Mallen JR, Roberts DS. SCUBA Medicine for Otolaryngologists: Part II. Diagnostic, Treatment, and Dive Fitness Recommendations. Laryngoscope. 2020 Jan;130(1):59-64. doi: 10.1002/lary.27874. Epub 2019 Feb 18. PMID: 30776095

25. Merchant S N, McKenna M J, Rosowski J J. Current status and future challenges of tympanoplasty.Eur Arch Otorhinolaryngol 1998; 255(5): 221-8

26. Merchant S N, Ravicz M E, Voss S E, Peake W T, Rosowski J J. Toynbee Memorial Lecture 1997. Middle ear mechanics in normal, diseased and reconstructed ears. J Laryngol Otol 1998; 112(8): 715-31

27. Meyer MF, Boor M, Jansen S, Pracht ED, Felsch M, Klünter HD, Hüttenbrink K-B, Beutner D, Grosheva M. Influence of repetitive diving in saltwater on pressure equalization and Eustachian tube function in recreational scuba divers. Diving and Hyperbaric Medicine. 2017 December;47(4):216-222. doi10.28920/dhm47.4.216-222.

28. Monnot D, Michot T, Dugrenot E, Guerrero F, Lafère P. A survey of scuba diving-related injuries and outcomes among French recreational divers. Diving and Hyperbaric Medicine. 2019 June 30;49(2):96–106. doi: 10.28920/dhm49.96-106. PMID: 31177515.

29. Murrison A W, Smith D J, Francis T J R, Counter R T. Maxillary sinus barotrauma with fifth cranial nerve involvement. J Laryngol Otol 1991; 105: 217-9

30. Nofz L, Porrett J, Yii N, de Alwis N. Diving-related otological injuries: Initial assessment and management. Aust J Gen Pract. 2020 Aug;49(8):500-504. doi: 10.31128/AJGP-01-20-5191. PMID: 32738862

31. Parell G J, Becker G D. Neurological Consequences of Scuba Diving with Chronic Sinusitis. Laryngoscope 2000; 110: 1358-60

32. Pau H W. Inner ear damage in TORP-operated ears: an experimental study on the danger from environmental air pressure changes. Ann Otol Rhinol Laryngol 1000; 108(8): 745-9

33. Peifer K J. Tinnitus, aetiology and management. Clin Geriatric Med 1999; 15(1): 193-204

34. Pulec J L, Deguine C. Extensive tympanosclerosis with a fixed malleus. Ear Nose Throat J 1999; 78(5): 326

35. Richard L, Bouletreau P, Cantaloube D. An unusual fracture of the orbital floor. Rev Stomatol Chir Maxillofac 1999; 100(6): 315-8 Roydhouse N. Underwater Ear and Nose Care. Best Publishing Co 1993; Flagstaff, AZ, USA Roydhouse N. Round window membrane rupture in scuba divers. SPUMS J 1997; 27(3): 148-51

36. Rozycki SW, Brown MJ, Camacho M. Inner ear barotrauma in divers: an evidence-based tool for evaluation and treatment Diving Hyperb Med 2018 Sep 30;48(3):186-193. doi: 10.28920/dhm48.3.186-193. PMID: 30199891 PMCID: PMC6205852

37. Sames C, Gorman DF, Mitchell SJ, Zhou L, The impact of diving on hearing: a 10-25 year audit of New Zealand professional divers. Diving and Hyperbaric Medicine, 01 Mar 2019, 49(1):2-8

38. Sheridan M F, Hetherington H H, Hull J J. Inner ear barotrauma from scuba diving. Ear Nose Throat J 1999; 78(3): 181,184, 186-7

39. Shurpak A, Doweck I, Gremberg R, Gordon C R, Spitzer O, Melamed Y, Meyer W. Diving related Inner Ear Injuries. Laryngoscope 1991; 101: 173-9Taylor DM, Lippmann J, Smith D. The absence of hearing loss in otologically asymptomatic recreational scuba divers. Undersea Hyperb Med. 2006 Mar-Apr;33(2):135-41.

40. St Leger Dowse M, Waterman MK, Jones R, Smerdon GR. Aural health awareness and incident prevention in UK scuba divers. Diving Hyperb Med. 2022 Mar 31;52(1):22-26. doi: 10.28920/dhm52.1.22-26. PMID: 35313369; PMCID: PMC9177430.

41. Wingelaar TT, Endert EL, Hoencamp R, van Ooij PJAM, van Hulst RA. Longitudinal screening of hearing threshold in navy divers: is diving really a hazard? Diving and Hyperbaric Medicine. 2019 December 20;49(4):283–290. doi: 10.28920/dhm49.4.283-290. PMID: 31828747.

# 12 Gastrointestinal Diseases

## POINTS TO PONDER

- Gastrointestinal barotrauma can be caused by gas distending the intestines on the ascent. Symptoms include abdominal pain and discomfort, bloated sensations, nausea, vomiting and eructation during or following ascent. It can be caused by:
  - » Any condition that traps gas in any part of the intestine. If gas moves into that area during a dive and is trapped whilst the diver makes an ascent, distension will occur.
  - » Swallowing air during a dive may fill the stomach which becomes distended on the ascent. It can occur with anxiety and with equalising techniques where swallowing is applied, e.g., Toynbee manoeuvre. If excessive, a rupture of the stomach may occur.
  - » Drinking gaseous drinks before diving.
  - » Head-down positions, especially when combined with Valsalva manoeuvres, encourage air to move more easily up the oesophagus into the stomach.
- Vomiting whilst underwater can clog the regulator mechanism, creating a free flow. The spasm of the chest and abdominal walls can splint the lungs, inhibit exhalation and predispose to pulmonary barotrauma. There is often a reflex inspiration after vomiting with the risk of aspiration of vomit and water (Novomesky).
- Any condition which causes acute, disabling, colicky pain whilst diving is dangerous.

## OESOPHAGEAL CONDITIONS

### Achalasia

- This causes ineffective and later absent peristalsis in the body of the oesophagus with loss of coordinated relaxation of the lower oesophageal sphincter. Atony and dilation of the lower oesophagus occur.

Consider the risk of regurgitation, oesophageal spasm or even tracheal aspiration by pooled secretions and food in the lower oesophagus when diving in head-down positions (a plausible, regular and moderate risk).

**The risk may be removed by avoiding head-down positions.**

## Gastro-Oesophageal Reflux Disease (GORD)

- A common condition from the mild occasional "heartburn" to the severe disabling ulcerative oesophagus.
- Severe cases may suffer sudden incapacitating chest or epigastric pain. Treatment may include proton pump inhibitors and/or cisapride.
- Failed conservative treatment may lead to a fundoplication.

Consider the risks of regurgitation, oesophageal spasm and even tracheal aspiration by refluxing gastric contents when diving in a head-down position.

**This risk may be reduced by avoiding head-down positions.**

**We discourage any diver with severe symptoms to dive until improved.**

## Hiatus Hernia

- Part of the stomach herniates through the diaphragm. It may herniate directly (sliding) or the stomach may push up beside the oesophagus (para-oesophageal). It may make the cardiac sphincter incompetent and be associated with gastro-oesophageal reflux.
- A non-symptomatic sliding hiatus hernia is of no consequence in diving.
- An incarcerated sliding or para-oesophageal hernia could trap air and become overdistended with the danger of rupture.
- After corrective surgery by fundoplication, the stomach can suffer "gas bloat" syndrome with gaseous distension of the stomach.
- A case of diaphragmatic rupture has been attributed to such distension during a dive (Hayden).

Consider the risk of trapping air in an incarcerated sliding or any para-oesophageal hernia causing severe pain and even rupture of the hernia or diaphragm (a possible, rare and major risk).

**The risk may be reduced by avoiding head-down positions.**

**We would not recommend anyone with a para-oesophageal hernia, repaired or otherwise to dive.**

## Oesophageal Diverticula

- The diverticulum accumulates secretions and food particles.

Consider the risk of regurgitation, oesophageal spasm or even tracheal aspiration by pooled secretions and food when diving in head-down positions,(a plausible, regular and moderate risk).

**The risk may be removed by surgical correction of thediverticulum**

**We would not recommend diving unless the diverticulum was very small.**

## Oesophageal Varices

- The varices are usually a serious complication of cirrhosis and portal hypertension.
- While diving immersion will cause a shunting of blood from the periphery to the central circulation. This will engorge the gastrointestinal blood volume. People with chronic portal hypertension have an abnormal response to increased central venous pressure, exacerbating the increased central blood volume and producing further gastrointestinal vascular engorgement.
- Further, on the ascent, the expansion of intra-luminal gastrointestinal gas may engorge the portal venous circulation (Nguyen). One case of massive variceal bleeding provoked by scuba diving has been reported (Nguyen).

Consider the risk of the underlying cause of thevarices.

Consider the risk of provoking a variceal bleed (a plausible, rare and major risk).

**We would not recommend diving to anyone with oesophageal varices.**

### Primary Oesophageal Motility Disorders

- A syndrome of painful dysphagia marked by regurgitation and choking, often precipitated by cold liquids.

Consider the risk of regurgitation and oesophageal spasm during diving (a possible, remote and moderate risk).

**The risk may be reduced by avoiding head-down positions.**

### Scleroderma of the Oesophagus

- Increased collagen and fibrosis in the lower two-thirds of the oesophagus cause hypomobility with loss of function causing a gastro-reflux.

Consider the risk of the other systems involved in the condition.

Consider the risks of regurgitation, oesophageal spasm and even tracheal aspiration by refluxing gastric contents when diving in a head-down position.

**The risk may be reduced by avoiding head-down positions.**

**We would not recommend diving with anyone with this condition.**

## GASTRIC CONDITIONS

### Bariatric Surgery

Roux-en-Y surgery, Gastric sleeve, Gastric banding (Lap banding), Gastric balloon

- These procedures have become far more commonplace for effective and sustainable weight loss in the past 20 years.
- The general fitness of the obese diver should be considered – (see the section dedicated to obesity)
- Long-term complications include dumping syndrome (see below), chronic vomiting and malnutrition should be discussed.
- The gastric bands and balloons are filled with saline and not subject to barotrauma.
- Acid reflux can be aggravated especially on the ascent.

**If fit and unaffected by disabling side effects, diving is recommended.**

### Gastric Outlet Obstruction/Pyloric Stenosis

- This is usually a late complication of duodenal ulceration. It has become rare since the efficiency of medication and eradication of Helicobacter pylori.
- Frequent vomiting and gastric distension are common symptoms.
- Metabolic disturbances abound.
- Surgery is the only treatment.

Consider the risk of air trapping in the stomach and gastrointestinal barotrauma.

**The patient is usually unwell and would not want to dive.**

## Partial Afferent Loop Obstruction

- This may occur in patients with a sub-total gastrectomy and a gastro-jejunostomy (Roux-en-Y and Bilroth II procedures). The afferent loop may become dilated with pancreatic and biliary secretions, especially if there is a stenosis.
- The main symptom is abdominal pain. Gas could pass into the loop and dilate on ascent causing distension

Consider the risk of severe abdominal pain by gas expanding in the loop on the ascent (a possible, rare and moderate risk).

**The diver should be warned of the potential problems so that if symptoms are caused, they can decide on their future diving.**

## Peptic Ulceration/Duodenal Ulcer, Gastric Ulcer

The main symptom is epigastric pain, which can be acute and disabling. Insidious bleeding can cause anaemia.

- Most people with this condition will have had an endoscopy and be on drug treatment.

Consider the risk of acute disabling abdominal pain whilst diving.

**We recommend diving as long as symptoms are controlled by anti-ulcer medication.**

## Post-Gastrectomy Syndromes

Dumping Syndrome, Afferent Loop Syndrome, Small stomach syndrome

- In severe cases, it can be associated with vomiting, weakness, faintness, palpitations, flushing, and lassitude after meals.

Consider the risk of suddenly feeling faint and weak during a dive.

**The risk may be reduced by not diving after meals when the symptoms are expected.**

## Late Dumping syndrome

- Symptoms include diaphoresis, palpitations, lassitude, mental confusion and even loss of consciousness 1/2 to 3 hours after a meal.

Consider the risk of sudden weakness and confusion or even loss of consciousness whilst diving.

**The risk may be reduced by not diving ½ to 3 hours after a meal and having some sweet supplements before diving.**

## Recurrent Vomiting

e.g., Cyclical Vomiting, Abdominal Migraine, Psychogenic Vomiting, Bulimia

- Occurs usually in young adults with a history of recurrent vomiting. If frequent it can cause dehydration and metabolic problems.
- Beware of undiagnosed pathology.

Consider the risks of uncontrolled vomiting underwater.

# CONDITIONS OF SMALL AND LARGE INTESTINES AND ASSOCIATED ORGANS

## Colostomy and Ileostomy

- The normal colostomy and ileostomy stomas are of no concern whilst diving.
- It is recommended to apply a fresh bag before a dive.
- A "continent" ileostomy e.g., Koch Pouch, can trap air with possible distension and rupture on the ascent.

Consider the risk of distension and rupture of a continent ileostomy (a possible, rare and major risk).

## Diverticular Disease of the large intestine

- These small diverticuli are very common and are freely communicating with the colon. They have no relevance to diving unless they become acutely inflamed and cause colicky lower abdominal pains and fever.

## Gallstones

- Gallstones are usually symptomless.
- If they block or move within the duct, they can cause biliary colic with sudden and severe colicky pains, vomiting and nausea.

Consider the risk of biliary colic occurring whilst diving causing sudden incapacitation.

**We advise anyone who has had recent biliary colic to delay diving until it has been surgically treated.**

## Inflammatory Bowel Disease (IBD)

Crohn's Disease, Ulcerative Colitis, Regional Colitis

- These are usually chronic illnesses with generalised ill health and continuous or intermittent diarrhoea. Other symptoms include fevers, abdominal pain, aphthous ulcers and weight loss. They commonly affect the 20 - 40 year age group.
- Complications include anaemia, electrolyte imbalance and dehydration producing lethargy and weakness.
- There may be long periods of remission.
- Long-term treatment may include TNF inhibitors, immunosuppressants and sulphasalazine, which itself can cause nausea and vomiting. Rarely it causes haematological disorders and fibrosing alveolitis.
- Corticosteroids may also need to be given long-term, which can have disabling side effects.

Consider the risk of diving whilst debilitated with chronic diarrhoea.

Consider the risk of the side effects of the treatment.

**We recommend diving if they are in remission or if their symptoms are mild and controlled. Most people with inflammatory bowel disease have a wide understanding of their condition and physical capabilities.**

## Small Bowel Obstruction

- Usually associated with peritoneal adhesions following previous abdominal surgery.
- It can cause sudden abdominal colicky and disabling pains.

Consider the risk of sudden disabling pain whilst diving.

## Pancreatitis – chronic or recurring

- This is characterised by chronic ill health, recurrent abdominal pains, weight loss and diabetes mellitus.
- It is sometimes caused by alcohol abuse.

Consider the risk of diving whilst debilitated causing reduced exercise tolerance and easy fatigue.

Consider the risk of any complications such as diabetes.

Consider the risk of sudden incapacitating pain whilst diving.

**We would not recommend anyone with this condition to dive.**

## FURTHER READING:


1. Edmonds C. Diving is a pain in the Gut (letter). SPUMS J 1995; 25(2): 67-8
2. Hunter J D, Roobottom C A, Bryson P J, Brown C. Conservative management of gastric rupture following scuba diving. J Accid Emerg Med 1998; 15(2): 116-7
3. Hayden J D, Davies J B, Martin I G. Diaphragmatic rupture from gastrointestinal barotrauma in a scuba diver. Br J Sports Med 1998; 32 (1): 75-6
4. Molenat F A, Boussuges A H. Rupture of the stomach complicating diving accidents. Undersea Hyperbar Med 1995; 22(1): 87-96
5. Novomeský F, Janík M, Hájek M, Krajčovič J, Straka L. Vomiting and aspiration of gastric contents: a possible life-threatening combination in underwater diving. Diving Hyperb Med. 2018 Mar 31;48(1):36-39. oi: 10.28920/dhm48.1.36-39. PMID: 29557100
6. Novomeský F, Krajcovic J, Stuller F. Vomitus as a cause of fatal diving accident of a commercial diver. Soud Lek. 2010 Jan;55(1):5-7.
7. Nguyen M H, Ernsting K S, Proctor D D. Massive variceal bleeding caused by scuba diving. Am J Gastroenteral 2000; 95(12): 3677-8
8. Paramsothy M, Goh K L, Kannan P. Esophageal motility disorders: rapid functional diagnosis using computerised radionuclide oesophagal transit study. Singapore Med J 1995; 26(3): 309-13
9. Titu LV, Laden G, Purdy G, Wedgwood. Gastric barotrauma in a scuba diver: report of a case. Surg Today. 2003;33(4):299-301.
10. Vuilleumier H, Vouillamoz D, Cuttat J F. Gastric rupture secondary to barotrauma in the framework of a diving accident. Apropos of a case report and literature review. Swiss Surg 1995; (5): 226-9
11. Yeung P, Crowe P, Bennett M. Barogenic rupture of the stomach: a case for non-operative management. Aust N Z J Surg 1998; 68(1): 76-7

# 13 Haematological Diseases

## POINTS TO PONDER

- The oxygen-carrying capacity of the blood is dependent on the type and level of the haemoglobin. Any reduction in the amount of oxygen that can be transported by the blood will cause easy fatigue and reduced exercise tolerance. Severe reductions will result in breathlessness and heart failure.
- Keep into consideration that the oxygen partial pressure increases with depth, thus offsetting the decrease in haemoglobin.

## ABNORMAL RED CELLS

Congenital/Spherocytosis, Elliptocytosis, Ovalocytosis, Stomatocytosis

- Usually, cause mild anaemia but the haemoglobin can be normal.
- Elevated oxygen partial pressure can precipitate haemolysis in hereditary spherocytosis and glucose-6-phosphate dehydrogenase deficiency.

Consider the risk of severe anaemia causing fatigue and reduced exercise tolerance.

**This risk may be reduced if the anaemia is long-standing and within 2g/L of normal.**

**We would advise individuals with hereditary spherocytosis and glucose-6-phosphate dehydrogenase deficiency to avoid high partial pressures of oxygen, e.g., in deep diving and accelerated decompression with 100% oxygen.**

## ANAEMIA

- The cause of the low haemoglobin needs to be determined and assessed.
- Anaemia will reduce the oxygen-carrying capacity of the blood causing faintness, fatigue, tiredness, breathlessness and reduced exercise tolerance.
- Angina, heart failure and confusion can be provoked.
- The severity and longevity of the anaemia will determine to what degree the anaemia is disabling.

Consider the risk of the underlying cause of the anaemia.

Consider the risk of severe anaemia causing faintness, fatigue and reduced exercise tolerance.

**This risk may be reduced if the anaemia is long-standing and within 2g/L of normal.**

## BLEEDING DISORDERS

e.g., Haemophilia, von Willebrand's disease, thrombocytopenia, anticoagulant therapy with coumarins or factor Xa inhibitors

- Barotrauma of any type may cause bleeding, either from a negative pressure causing petechiae and eventually frank haemorrhage from superficial blood vessels e.g., in the mucosa of the middle ear or sinuses, or from the tearing of overstretched tissues e.g., in the lung when over-expanded.
- Neurological decompression illness (especially of the spinal cord) may be associated with haemorrhage within the neural tissue.
- Inner ear decompression illness is associated with haemorrhage within the cochlea.

Consider the risk of a minor bleed e.g., from minor barotrauma, all the way to a major bleed.

**This risk may be reduced by taking special care in equalizing the middle ear and ascending very slowly and limiting the depth and frequency of diving.**

**We strongly discourage anyone with bleeding disorders from diving in view of the risk of bleeding and aggravating the clinical situation if neurological DCI were to develop.**

## POLYCYTHAEMIA

Polycythaemia Rubra Vera (PRV), Polycythaemia Vera (PV)

- Excess red cells in circulation can be associated with living at high altitudes. More often it is a symptom of serious disease, either primary (true polycythaemia vera, a myeloproliferative disorder) or secondary e.g., heavy smoking, sleep apnoea, chronic obstructive pulmonary disease (COPD) causing chronic hypoxia.
- The increased red cell density will impair tissue perfusion perhaps predisposing to decompression illness (DCI) and aggravate any hypercoagulability caused by DCI in view of hyperviscosity.
- The expanded blood volume causes increased peripheral resistance, reduced cardiac output and exercise tolerance.
- The spleen is frequently massively enlarged, being vulnerable to rupture from trauma from weight belts and diving gear or just entering or exiting rough water.

Consider the risk of any underlying disease.

Consider the risk of reduced exercise tolerance.

Consider the risk of increased incidence of decompression illness.

Consider the risk of massive splenomegaly.

**We do not recommend anyone with this condition to dive, except those with polycythaemia vera who have no end-organ damage or complications and are being successfully treated and maintaining a normal packed red cell volume (PCV).**

## SICKLE CELL DISEASE

- This inherited disorder causes the production of Haemoglobin S (HbS).
- The homozygote (SS) has sickle cell anaemia.
- The heterozygote (AS) has sickle cell trait.

## Sickle Cell Anaemia

- The sickle-shaped red blood cells are fragile and haemolyse, causing severe anaemia. They are also more rigid and tend to obstruct capillary blood flow, causing infarction and local hypoxia.
- Hypoxia, cold, dehydration and even muscular exertion can cause excessive sickling and exacerbate a sickle cell crisis with thrombosis, often in the bones, causing severe bone pain and even marrow aplasia. A crisis can mimic an acute abdomen or pneumonia and even produce a convulsion.
- Recurrent vaso-occlusive insults can impair pulmonary function and can cause intrapulmonary arterial venous shunting. This could reduce the effectiveness of the pulmonary vascular filter and predispose to decompression illness. Other chronic complications include renal failure, bone necrosis, osteomyelitis and leg ulcers.
- Individuals are more susceptible to convulsions, possibly due to silent CNS infarction and they are also very susceptible to oxygen-induced seizures.

Consider the risk of severe anaemia causing fatigue and reduced exercise tolerance.

Consider the risk of cold, muscular activity and dehydration precipitating a crisis whilst diving.

Consider the risk of complications arising.

**We would not recommend anyone with homozygous sickle cell disease to dive.**

## Sickle Cell Trait

- The heterozygote form of sickle cell disease has a very silent clinical course.
- It occurs in 8.7% of African Americans in the USA and confers a protective advantage against malaria infection.

**There seems to be no risk associated with the trait for diving.**

# THALASSAEMIA

- This is a deficiency of the synthesis of the alpha or beta chains of haemoglobin is seen frequently in people originating from the Middle and Far East and the Mediterranean.
- ß thalassemia major
- This is the homozygote form and results in severe hypochromic and haemolytic anaemia that presents in early life as failure to thrive.
- Infants who survive may develop the endocrine disease, liver disease and cardiac toxicity from iron overload and bony deformities.
- Treatment is improving with adequate transfusion, iron chelation therapy and allogeneic bone marrow transplantation.

Consider the risk of anaemia causing fatigue and reduced exercise tolerance.

Consider the risk of complications commonly associated with this condition.

**We would not recommend anyone with thalassemia major to dive.**

## ß thalassemia minor

- The heterozygote form is usually asymptomatic. It can cause mild hypochromic, microcytic anaemia.

Consider the risk of anaemia causing fatigue and reduced exercise tolerance.

**The risk may be reduced if the anaemia is long-standing and within 2g/L of normal.**

**If they are symptomless and the haemoglobin is near normal, we will recommend diving.**

# FURTHER READING:

1. Vigilante J A, Di George NW. Sickle cell trait and diving: review and recommendations. Undersea Hyperb Med May-Jun 2014;41(3):223-8.

# Infectious Diseases

# 14

## POINTS TO PONDER

There are two important risks to consider with any infectious disease – the risk associated with the disease itself and the risk to which other divers may be exposed:

- The disease itself:
  - » Many infectious diseases are associated with disabling symptoms such as fatigue, fever, tiredness, vomiting and dehydration.
  - » Most infectious diseases are self-limiting and will only disable a diver for a short period.
  - » Many chronic diseases are completely symptom-free for many years. Some infections are now treated prophylactically before any disability occurs e.g., HIV. The drugs used may have adverse drug reactions.
- The risk of transmitting the disease:
  - » The main method of transfer of infection between divers used to be "buddy breathing", where a regulator was transferred between two divers' mouths. Although this emergency procedure was rarely used whilst actually diving, it was a compulsory lesson during all diving courses.
  - » This practice has now largely ceased and all divers should be equipped with a second (octopus) regulator for emergency out-of-air situations.
  - » Certain infectious diseases merit specific mention:

## HIV INFECTION

- The HIV virus is not easily transmitted. It requires the transmission of infected blood or body fluid across the skin/mucous membrane barrier, usually by sharing contaminated needles or anal/ vaginal intercourse.
- The concentration of the virus in the saliva is very low compared to blood and semen. There is no confirmed case of transmission via contaminated saliva.
- The virus is not tolerant of conditions outside the body.

## HIV positive individuals

- People who are HIV positive are usually well. Many will be taking a combination of viral suppression anti-retroviral drugs to reduce the viral load, hopefully to undetectable levels.
- People who are HIV positive seem to suffer more adverse drug reactions (ADR) than the normal population e.g., HIV patients have a 50% incidence of ADRs to trimethoprim-sulphamethoxazole compared to a 10% incidence in the general population.
- It has been postulated that intravascular bubbles formed during dives could compromise the blood-brain barrier allowing premature transmission of the virus to the brain.
- Consider the risk of premature transmission of the virus to the brain (a possible, rare and moderate risk).

Consider the risk of side effects of anti-retroviral drugs and other drugs taken for incidental problems.

**If the diver is well and has no disabling or ambiguous side effects from their medication that could be confused with decompression illness, we would recommend diving.**

## AIDS-related complex (ARC)

- As the CD4 cell count falls <300, symptoms such as persistent oral candidiasis, shingles, chronic fatigue, idiopathic thrombocytopenia, fever and weight loss develop.

Consider the risk of these debilitating symptoms on the diver's stamina and exercise tolerance.

## AIDS / Acquired Immune Deficiency Syndrome

- AIDS patients suffer opportunistic infections and malignancies e.g., P. jirovecii pneumonia, toxoplasmosis encephalitis, cytomegalic infection tuberculosis, lymphoma and Kaposi's sarcoma.
- In addition to taking antiretroviral drugs, they may also be taking other drugs against these infections.

Consider pulmonary pathology which could predispose to pulmonary barotrauma.

Consider the risk of each infection or malignancy.

Consider the risk of such debilitating conditions reducing the diver's stamina and exercise tolerance.

**We would not recommend anyone with ARC or AIDS to dive.**

# HEPATITIS

These viral infections that target the liver will commonly cause fatigue, nausea, anorexia and jaundice.

## Hepatitis A

- This acute form is commonly acquired in travellers. It is transmitted by the faecal/oral route, often from a contaminated water supply. The disease is transmissible for a variable period before and after the acute onset of symptoms.
- The incubation period is 15-50 days so most divers will be back home from their diving holiday before symptoms appear.
- It may cause very severe fatigue, abdominal pains, vomiting and jaundice. Vaccination is available.

Consider the risk of fatigue reducing stamina and exercise tolerance.

Consider the risk of transmission to fellow divers.

**We would not recommend diving until all symptoms have settled.**

**If using rented regulators or travelling overseas, we would recommend routine active immunization to the divers.**

## Hepatitis B

- The acute form is acquired by the transmission of blood or body fluids across the skin/mucous membrane barrier usually by sharing needles or anal/vaginal sex. It is a much more virulent virus than the HIV virus and can remain viable outside the body for longer periods. However, the risk of transmission in the diving environment between divers is very small.
- Symptoms also include arthralgia and urticaria.
- Chronic active hepatitis occurs in 1-3% of cases. Continued abnormal liver function tests are associated with anorexia, weight loss and fatigue. Complications include cirrhosis and hepato- cellular cancer.
- 5-10% of cases become carriers who, although clinically well, shed the virus in their body fluids.
- Vaccination is available.

Consider the risk of fatigue reducing stamina and exercise tolerance.

**We would not recommend diving until all symptoms had settled.**

**We would recommend routine immunisation to the divers.**

## Hepatitis C

- This is an ever-increasing problem despite recent public health strategies which have helped control the HIV epidemic. Most cases are not diagnosed for many years after infection.
- It is transmitted by blood transfusion and injecting drugs. There is virtually no risk of transmission in the diving environment between divers.
- About 80% of those infected develop chronic liver disease, many are asymptomatic but many suffer fatigue. Long-term complications include cirrhosis (10-20%) and hepatocellular cancer (5%). Although there is no vaccine for Hepatitis C, anti-viral treatment can reduce the viral load to undetectable levels. The virus is considered cured when it is not detected 12 weeks after treatment is completed.

Consider the risk of fatigue reducing stamina and exercise tolerance.

Consider the risk of any medication.

**If the diver is symptom-free and has no disabling adverse drug reactions, we would recommend diving.**

## Hepatitis D

- This is an incomplete RNA virus that only exists in the presence of hepatitis B and is spread by the same routes. It should be considered in the same way.
- There is no vaccination available.

## Hepatitis E

- This is similar to hepatitis A and is spread by the same routes. It should be considered in the same way.
- There is no vaccination available.

## MALARIA

- This is the most common infection in the world. There are several protozoal plasmodia and their virulence influences the severity, prophylaxis and treatment of the disease. Its incubation period is 1-6 weeks.
- Symptoms are characterized by rigors, fever, weakness, jaundice and anaemia, but early symptoms can be just like the "flu" and can be confused with symptoms of decompression illness (DCI).

Consider the risk of reduced stamina and exercise tolerance.

**We would not recommend anyone with acute malaria to dive.**

**We reinforce all the methods of avoiding malaria as well as recommending antimalarial prophylaxis when travelling to malaria areas.**

**Mefloquine prophylaxis is contra-indicated in divers, due to its known psychiatric adverse effects.**

## FURTHER READING:

1. Petersen K, Regis DP. Safety of antimalarial medications for use while scuba diving in malaria Endemic Regions. Trop Dis Travel Med Vaccines. 2016 Oct 11;2:23. doi: 10.1186/s40794-016-0041-x. PMID: 28883967; PMCID: PMC5530948.
2. Pougnet R, Pougnet L, Henckes A, Allio I, Lucas D, Dewitte JD, Loddé B. Infectious diseases affecting occupational divers: a review of 2017 literature. Int Marit Health. 2018;69(3):176-180. doi: 10.5603/IMH.2018.0028. PMID: 30270418.
3. Rodrigues KMP, Moreira BM. Preventing diseases in round-the-world travellers: a contemporary challenge for travel medicine advice. Rev Soc Bras Med Trop. 2018 Mar-Apr;51(2):125-132. doi: 10.1590/0037-8682-0418-2017. PMID: 29768543.

# Malignant Diseases 15

## POINTS TO PONDER

- Each case involving cancer and malignancy must be assessed on an individual basis, taking into consideration the huge variety of about 200 tumour types affecting 60 organs in the human body, with neoplasm/tumour site, grade, degree of invasiveness, distant spread and systemic effects from the tumour or the treatment entertained from for management of the tumour itself.
- The risks should be assessed on different levels:

Consider the risk of the primary malignancy.

Common symptoms of malignant disease include weakness, fatigue, lethargy, loss of appetite and weight loss.

Consider the risk of complications of the primary malignancy.

These include depressive illness, secondary bleeding tendencies, anaemia, pulmonary infiltrates, myopathies and neuropathies, pulmonary and pericardial effusions, ascites, opportunistic infections and mass effects.

Consider the risk of the effects and complications of secondary deposits, e.g. metastases in the brain or lung predisposing to generalized convulsions or pulmonary barotrauma of ascent with arterial gas embolism, respectively.

Consider the risks of the effects of treatment, including:

- The debilitating effects of recent surgery.
- The side-effects of cytotoxic drugs, especially nausea, vomiting, bleeding disorders, pulmonary pneumonitis and fibrosis.
- The very late complications of radiotherapy include fibrosis of soft tissues and lungs within the radiation field, coronary artery disease, thyroid dysfunction and pancytopenia.

Consider the prognosis of the condition. The diver may have a predicted short time to dive with a brief window of opportunity to be active.

Consider the benefit of doing an activity that would increase the quality of life and rehabilitation of the individual.

We have occasionally been confronted by terminally ill divers who want to accept foolhardy risks because of their short life expectancy. This must be confronted and strongly discouraged to protect not only the diver but, as importantly, the others involved in the dive; the dive buddies, dive and boat staff and other divers participating in the dive.

## FURTHER READING:

1. Douglas J D. Palliative care and Sports Medicine: Can the decision-making process ever overlap? Br J Sports Med 1999; 33(4): 238

# Mental Health Issues

# 16

## POINTS TO PONDER

- Scuba diving is both physically and cognitively demanding. It requires clear thinking and controlled reactions allowing planning, problem-solving and decision-making. Any condition that will significantly reduce awareness, attention and concentration or increase impulsiveness or uncertainty will compromise diving safety.
- Mental health conditions, especially depression and anxiety, affect about 20% of the Australian population (Australian Bureau of Statistics). This statistic was pre-COVID-19.
- The stigma of mental health conditions encourages many divers to hide their symptoms and /or medications in fear of adverse judgement and/or exclusion from diving (St Leger Dowse).
- Few divers perceived their mental health issues to affect their ability to dive. Over 90% who took medications considered they did not have any effect on their ability to dive
- Many psychiatric disorders are relapsing and recurring. If a diver is assessed in a period of quiescence and advised that the risk is acceptable, it is of concern that if the condition relapses, the diver's insight might be impaired and a new risk assessment avoided.
- Many perceive scuba diving to be of benefit to their mental health. The relaxation of being in a 'blue space', the mindfulness whilst diving, being weightless (the floatation effect), the exercise and socialization have all been identified to be beneficial.

## ANXIETY

Chronic anxiety disorder, generalized anxiety disorder (GAD)

- Anxiety is a normal human emotion and part of a normal response to a new experience or challenge (like learning to dive). Sufferers of an anxiety disorder, however, feel apprehension and dread without an identifiable stimulus or excessive symptoms. Even the fear of an anxiety attack itself can induce anxiety.
- Thirteen percent of Australians suffer from anxiety disorders (Australian Bureau of Statistics).
- Symptoms include fatigue, irritability, poor concentration and insomnia. Physical effects include hyperventilation, sweating, faintness, palpitations, nausea, and diarrhoea.
- Anxiety may quickly lead to paralysis of thinking and panic, with a surge of fear which underwater can result in an uncontrolled ascent and pulmonary barotrauma. It has been suggested that divers with elevated levels of trait anxiety

may be more prone to panic (Morgan).

- Treatment has changed over the past 20 years. Benzodiazepines are rarely used except in acute situations. Selective serotonin reuptake inhibitors (SSRIs) are most commonly used. Side effects include insomnia, nausea, vomiting, dry mouth and agitation.

Consider the risk of symptoms of acute anxiety occurring whilst diving, clouding thinking and even leading to panic, unable to help self or buddy (a plausible, regular and major risk).

Consider the risk of any medication being taken.

**These risks can be minimized by avoiding diving for three months after commencement of a SSRI or when dosage is being reduced or withdrawn.**

**We would not recommend anyone with a recent history of any disabling symptoms of anxiety, especially hyperventilation, palpitations, nausea or panic attacks, or requiring high dosages of SSRIs or any dosage of a benzodiazepine medication to dive.**

## BIPOLAR DISORDER

Hypomania, Manic Depressive disorder, cyclothymic disorder

- There are four major categories of bipolar disorder: bipolar I disorder, bipolar II disorder, cyclothymic disorder, and bipolar disorder due to another medical or substance abuse disorder.
- People who have bipolar disorders have emotional states that are at times extreme and intense. The manic episodes of bipolar 1 are typically worse than the hypomanic episodes of bipolar 2.
- Although the symptoms come and go, bipolar disorder usually requires lifetime treatment and does not go away on its own. Depressive symptoms last for several weeks at a time whilst manic symptoms usually last for several days at a time. The mood is chaotic, not cyclical.
- In bipolar II, depression may be severe, but the highs are much milder and do not truly impair function. They may even make people more productive.
- Treatment for bipolar disorder is a combination of psychotherapy and medication. Most people take more than one drug, like a mood-stabilizing drug plus an antipsychotic, benzodiazepine, or antidepressant.
- Some of the commonly prescribed medications for bipolar disorder are the same as those prescribed for depression and anxiety. Others include lithium, valproate, lamotrigine, olanzapine and risperidone. Possible adverse side effects for divers include tiredness, dizziness, insomnia, nervousness, restlessness, nausea, vomiting, constipation, dry mouth, runny or stuffy nose, increased salivation, weight loss or gain, increased heart rate and low blood pressure.

Consider the risk of irresponsible actions with no insight or appreciation for the danger of the underwater environment (a possible, remote, major risk).

Consider the risk of depressive symptoms, lethargy, fatigue, poor concentration, and even suicidal ideation.

Consider the risk of any medication being taken.

**We would not recommend anyone with a recent history of mania to dive.**

**We would discourage anyone with a distant history of mania to dive.**

**If the condition is one of the milder classifications, well controlled over the past year and only one medication is taken with no adverse side effects then diving would be possible.**

## DEPRESSION

- Everyone gets low mood from time to time, but when it is accompanied by sleeping difficulties, feelings of hopelessness or worthlessness, fatigue, lack of motivation, motor retardation, poor concentration, lack of joy and even suicidal thoughts, it has become a clinical depression which can be disabling.
- Depression is common. It affects 10% of Australians.
- Many do not seek treatment from feelings of shame.
- Many divers will not declare an onset of symptoms for fear of being excluded from diving.
- Many people suffering a moderate to major depression will be on long-term medication.
- The commonest medications are the selective serotonin reuptake inhibitors (SSRIs), which usually are well tolerated but any antidepressant, especially the traditional older medications, can cause drowsiness, sleepiness, dry mouth and increase the danger of convulsions (Hill) and bleeding tendencies (especially if taking non-steroidal anti-inflammatory drugs (NSAIDs) or anticoagulants) (de Abajo, Cochran), especially if high dosages are needed.
- Reducing and/or withdrawing medication can aggravate a recurrence of symptoms.

Consider the risk of depression affecting the diver's ability to think and act decisively and safely whilst diving.

**This risk can be minimized by the diver waiting until any treatment has taken effect and their symptoms are well controlled. Divers who are suffering symptoms of depression seem to avoid diving, maybe from a lack of motivation (St Ledger Louse).**

Consider the risk of suicidal ideation whilst diving.

This should be directly asked.

Consider the risk of any medication being taken.

**This can be minimized if only one medication for depression has been taken compliantly for at least three months and no disabling adverse effects have occurred. Diving should be restricted to 18-20 meters (60-65 feet).**

**Moreover, diving should be stopped whilst the medication is withdrawn and/or replaced.**

Consider the risk of rare side effects of antidepressants, (seizures and bleeding tendencies)

**This can be avoided by not recommending diving to anyone with any history of epilepsy, no matter how long ago, nor for anyone taking anticoagulants, antiplatelet drugs or NSAIDs.**

## EATING DISORDERS

Anorexia nervosa / bulimia

- Pathologically excessive dieting can cause serious emaciation with significant mortality. Most people suffering from anorexia nervosa deny their problem and are brought to treatment by distraught parents or friends.
- It commonly involves an excessive preoccupation with food, feelings of inadequacy, anxiety, depression and suicide attempts.
- Poor nutrition causes fatigue, muscle wasting, hypothermia, and hypotension. The abuse of laxatives, diuretics and appetite suppressants or self-induced vomiting may cause disturbed blood chemistry, especially hypokalaemia.
- Cardiac dysrhythmias from hypokalaemia and prolonged Q-T interval are the commonest cause of death.
- The lack of body fat will predispose to hypothermia.

Consider the risk of muscle weakness and easy fatigue reducing stamina and exercise tolerance (a plausible, regular and moderate risk).

Consider the risk of dysrhythmias (a possible, rare and major risk).

Consider the risk of anxiety and depression reducing their ability to think and act quickly and safely during a dive.

**We would not recommend anyone with an ongoing eating disorder to dive. We would advise anyone who was in recovery to achieve normal nutrition, attain a body mass index (BMI) of 19 and gain some physical fitness and conditioning, especially by swimming.**

## PANIC ATTACKS

- These overwhelming and disabling feelings of terror and apprehension occur suddenly and often without warning.
- They are often accompanied by shortness of breath, hyperventilation, chest pains, palpitations and faintness.
- Symptoms can peak in 10 minutes and resolve in 20-30 minutes. Chest pains can initially be confused with myocardial infarction.
- Panic may provoke a rapid ascent to the surface with little regard for exhalation, predisposing to pulmonary barotrauma.
- The attacks can be aggravated by a certain situation e.g., a work, study or domestic situation. The fear of another attack can itself become the trigger.
- Higher than normal levels of carbon dioxide may be more likely to induce panic attacks in panic disorder patients (Matthew). Even after cessation of attacks, relapse is common.
- Treatment often includes an antidepressant medication.

Consider the risk of a panic attack occurring whilst diving (a plausible, regular and major risk).

**This risk may be reduced by delaying diving for an extended symptom-free period. Six months has been suggested.**

Consider the risks of any medication.

**These risks can be minimized by avoiding diving for three months after the commencement of an SSRI or when the dosage is being reduced or withdrawn.**

**We do not advise anyone who has had recent panic attacks (within six months) to dive. If there was an obvious aggravating factor which has been completely removed e.g., examinations, which are now over, or work stress resulting in a change of job, we would reduce this time to three months. If there is a long history of relapses we advise against further diving.**

## PHOBIAS

- These cause extreme distress when confronted with a phobic stimulus.
- A common reaction to a phobia is a panic attack. Underwater this may provoke a rapid ascent to the surface with little regard for exhalation. This is a recipe for pulmonary barotrauma of ascent leading to a cerebral arterial gas embolism (AGE), pneumothorax, or mediastinal or subcutaneous emphysema.
- Most phobias are unrelated to diving. Ones to consider include:

## Acrophobia

The fear of high places and falling. This can occasionally occur in very clear water when the diver perceives the danger of falling.

## Agoraphobia

The fear of wide-open spaces becomes relevant underwater for it is not uncommon whilst diving to be suspended in mid-water, unable to see the surface or the bottom. It can cause disorientation and feelings of isolation, the so-called "blue orb" or "blue dome" syndrome. It can be aggravated by nitrogen narcosis.

## Barophobia and Bathophobia

The fears of being crushed, and of sinking and depth, can occur if the diver is overweighted and sinks rapidly.

## Claustrophobia

The fear of enclosed spaces is even more relevant for divers for the underwater environment can become very "closed in". Water visibility can suddenly plummet as other divers kick up silt from the bottom. The sun going behind a cloud can create dark shadows. It becomes darker with depth. Claustrophobia can complicate treatment in hyperbaric chambers, especially small transportable chambers. Heavy sedation may be required.

## Elasmophobia

The fear of sharks is a very common fear for divers in waters where sharks swim and there is little to do except reassure the diver that left alone, they are usually harmless.

## Herpetophobia

The fear of snakes can be a problem when diving in areas inhabited by sea snakes which are curious creatures and like to follow and inspect the diver closely. Obviously, anyone with such a phobia should avoid such areas.

## Hydrophobia

It is not uncommon for a person to learn to dive to overcome their fear of open or deep water. A common fear, often bordering on phobia, especially of deep water is that of being pulled down by some underwater life form. Some people just had a bad experience whilst a child of being submerged whilst learning to swim. They feel that tackling the fear "full on" will help them to overcome it. Often it will, but the instructor needs to know their fears so they can be closely supervised and supported during their initial dives.

## Nyctophobia

The fear of darkness can suddenly intrude when clouds go behind the sun when at depth. Obviously, night, cave and wreck diving should be avoided.

## Pnigophobia

A fear of being unable to breathe, or of choking can easily emerge if there is any problem with the regulator and its airflow.

Consider the risk of the phobia inducing a panic attack whilst underwater leading to an uncontrolled ascent (a plausible, regular and major risk).

**This risk may be reduced by not diving in situations likely to encounter the stimulus, e.g., not diving in regions where sharks or sea snakes are found. The use of shot and anchor lines to aid descent and ascent will help orientate the diver against being lost and falling. Staying close to their buddy will also provide stability. Extra training with buoyancy control, avoiding murky water, night diving and deep diving may all be helpful.**

**We discuss with the diver whether they have a real phobia or just a fear. Many people are scared at the idea of seeing a shark underwater or are very uncomfortable if shut up in a cupboard but will not have a panic attack if it occurred. We would not recommend anyone with a true phobia which could occur during a dive to dive.**

## SCHIZOPHRENIA

- This psychosis affects 1% of the population.
- Symptoms include bizarre illusions, hallucinations, markedly illogical thinking and inappropriate reactions.
- Acute psychosis can mimic DCI (Hopkins).
- Treatment usually includes prophylactic antipsychotic drugs. Side effects include sedation, anticholinergic and extra-pyramidal effects (EPS). Newer antipsychotic drugs e.g., risperidone, olanzapine and clozapine, although having a lower incidence of EPS can cause sedation and orthostatic hypotension.
- There is a relapse rate of about 66% if antipsychotic drugs are withdrawn.
- A small number of patients with schizophrenia test positive for neuronal autoantibodies and respond to immunotherapies. These so-called 'autoimmune psychoses' may fully resolve. It is too early to know long-term recurrence (Pollak).

Consider the risk of delusions and hallucinations whilst diving.

Consider the risk of side effects of antipsychotic medication.

**We would not recommend anyone with a history of schizophrenia to dive.**

## POST TRAUMATIC STRESS DISORDER (PTSD)

- Post-traumatic stress disorder (PTSD) is a mental condition triggered by experiencing or witnessing a terrifying event or events e.g., war, rape, accident, assault, or natural disaster.
- Complex PTSD describes a more severe and long-term condition that can occur after prolonged and repeated trauma e.g., child abuse, or domestic violence.
- Symptoms are generally grouped into four types: intrusive (flashbacks), avoidance (hypervigilance), negative changes in thinking and mood (detachment, emotionally numb), and changes in physical and emotional reactions (irritability, insomnia). Symptoms can vary over time or vary from person to person.
- There are commonly co-morbidities e.g., depression, substance abuse
- Suicide is a common occurrence, especially in returned servicemen.
- Antidepressant medications, especially SSRIs, may be prescribed.
- Numerous anecdotal reports of PTSD sufferers gaining great symptomatic relief after scuba diving, especially when diving deeper than 20 m, have emerged (Diver Magazine, Hopkins medical blog).

Consider the risk of PTSD affecting the diver's ability to think and act decisively and safely whilst diving.

**This risk can be minimized by the diver waiting until any treatment has taken effect and their disabling symptoms are well controlled.**

Consider the risk of suicidal ideation whilst diving.

This should be directly asked.

Consider the risk of any medication being taken.

**This can be minimized if only one medication for PTSD has been taken compliantly for at least three months and no disabling adverse effects have occurred. Diving should be restricted to 18-20 meters (60-65 feet). Moreover, diving should be stopped whilst the medication is withdrawn and/or replaced.**

**We would not recommend anyone to dive who has symptoms that would compromise safety e.g., irrational actions, poor concentration and attention spans, and thoughts of self-harm. However, if well supervised (and many veteran organizations now have special diving programs) many PTSD sufferers may gain great benefits from diving.**

## FURTHER READING:


1. Australian Bureau of Statistics. (2018). National Health Survey: First Results 2017-18. Canberra: ABS
2. Carreno A, Gascon M, Vert C, Lloret J. The Beneficial Effects of Short-Term Exposure to Scuba Diving on Human Mental Health. Int J Environ Res Public Health. 2020 Oct 3;17(19):7238. doi: 10.3390/ijerph17197238. PMID: 33022983, PMCID: PMC7579011
3. Cochran KA, Cavallari LH, Shapiro NL, Bishop JR. Bleeding incidence with concomitant use of antidepressants and warfarin. Ther Drug Monit. 2011;33:433-8.12
4. de Abajo FJ, García Rodríguez A, Montero D. Antidepressant drugs: a potential new drug cause of upper gastrointestinal bleeding. Dig Liver Dis. 2000;32:455-7.10
5. Delphia B, Freed W. Depression: Its treatment and concerns regarding scuba diving. Alert Diver 1999; March/ April: 40-44
6. Diver magazine March 30th 2020 Diving and PTSD
7. Faraone SV, Sergeant J, Gillberg C, Biederman J. The worldwide prevalence of ADHD: is it an American condition? World Psychiatry. 2003;2:104–13. PMID: 16946911. PMCID: PMC1525089.
8. Hesdorffer DC, Ludvigsson P, Olafsson E, Gudmundsson G, Kjartansson O, Hauser WA. ADHD as a risk factor for incident unprovoked seizures and epilepsy in children. Arch Gen Psychiatry. 2004;61:731–6. doi: 10.1001/archpsyc.61.7.731. PMID: 15237085.
9. Hill T, Coupland C, Morriss R, Arthur A, Moore M, Hippisley-Cox J. Antidepressant use and risk of epilepsy and seizures in people aged 20 to 64 years: cohort study using a primary care database. BMC Psychiatry. 2015;15:315.
10. Hopkins R O, Weaver L K. Acute psychosis presenting as decompression illness. Undersea Hyper Med 2000; 27 (Supp): 27-8
11. Kaplan A, Garfinkel P. Medical Issues in Eating Disorders 1993. Brummel/Mazel, NY.
12. Keks N, Mazundar P, Shields R. New developments in schizophrenia. Aus Fam Phy 2000; 29(2): 129-36
13. Matthew R J, Wilson W H, Tant S. Responses to hypercarbia induced by azetazolamine in panic disorder patients. Am J Psychiatry 19889; 146(8): 996-1000
14. Morgan W P. Anxiety and panic in recreational scuba divers. Sports Med 1995; 20(6): 398-421

15. Morgan WP, Raglin JS, O Connor PJ. Trait anxiety predicts panic behaviour in beginning scuba students. Int J Sports Med. 2004;25:314-22.

16. Querido AL. Diving and antidepressants. Diving and Hyperbaric Medicine. 2017 December;47(4):253-256. doi10.28920/dhm47.4.253-256.

17. Querido AL, van Hulst RA. Diving and attention deficit hyperactivity disorder. Diving and Hyperbaric Medicine. 2019 March 31;49(1):41–47. doi: 10.28920/dhm49.1.41-47. PMID: 30856666.)

18. Pollak, Thomas A et al. Autoimmune psychosis: an international consensus on an approach to the diagnosis and management of psychosis of suspected autoimmune origin. The Lancet Psychiatry, 2020 Volume 7, Issue 1, 93 – 108. doi: https://doi org/10.1016/S2215-0366(10)30290-1

19. Schioberg- Schiegnitz S. Mental Fitness. Technical Diving for Sports Scuba Divers. SPUMS J 1996; 26(4): 277-80

20. St Leger Dowse M, Whalley B, Waterman MK, Conway RM, Smerdon GR. Diving and mental health: the potential benefits and risks from a survey of recreational scuba divers. Diving and Hyperbaric Medicine. 2019 December 20;49(4):291–297. doi: 10.28920/dhm49.4.291-297. PMID: 31828748.

21. Van Wijk CH, Martin JH, Firfirey N. Common mental health conditions among navy divers: a brief report. Diving Hyperb Med. 2020 Dec 20;50(4):417-420. doi: 10.28920/dhm50.4.417-420. PMID: 33325025, PMCID: PMC8026235

22. Yarbrough J. Anxiety: Is it a contraindication to diving? Alert Diver (SEAP Edition) 2001; Jan-Mar: 30-5

# Musculoskeletal Issues

# 17

## POINTS TO PONDER

- To obtain an open water diver certificate, most diving instructor agencies expect the diver to be able to put on all equipment, enter the water, swim, rescue a buddy, exit the water and remove equipment with no assistance.
- Kitting up is often undertaken in confined and cramped spaces, on pitching and rolling boat decks. Agility and stability of movement are required.
- Exiting the water can involve clambering into small boats, removing equipment in a swell before clambering up a pitching and rolling ladder or crawling and clambering over rocks or through surf.
- Diving tanks and weight belts are heavy and require some strength to manoeuvre and fit.
- Joint pain is a common symptom of decompression illness (DCI) so any pre-existing joint injury may be confusing.

## CERVICAL SPONDYLOSIS

- Kitting up may involve extreme movements of the neck such as looking around for a lost glove whilst sitting in a small boat, about to enter the water, in full gear and wearing a mask.
- Once in the water, there is usually no strain on the neck but, if positively buoyant, it may necessitate swimming with the back and neck hyperextended to keep the fins high and thrusting downwards. Clearing the mask may also often involve a full extension of the neck.
- Paraesthesia and numbness of the arms and hands, common complications of cervical spondylosis, may be confused with symptoms of decompression illness (DCI).

Consider the risk of aggravating neck pain from a pre-existing neck condition (a proven, regular and minor risk).

**This risk may be reduced by ensuring buoyancy and trim whilst underwater are adjusted to allow a neutral head position.**

Consider the risk of confusing paraesthesia and numbness of the upper limbs from a pre-existing neck condition with symptoms of DCI (a possible, remote and moderate risk).

**This risk may be reduced by limiting the depth and frequency of dives, ascending slowly and always incorporating a safety stop before surfacing.**

## LOW BACK PAIN

Lumbar Spondylosis, Prolapsed intervertebral disc (PID), Chronic low back pain

- Low back pain is a very common health problem worldwide and a major cause of disability. Chronic low back pain prevalence is estimated at 19.6% in those aged between 20 and 59 (Meucci).
- Many people suffering from low back pain are taking long-term daily narcotic analgesics.
- Diving involves lifting heavy equipment, kitting up in restricted, awkward spaces and pulling oneself onto boats, up ladders and over slippery rocks. Many dive trips involve bumpy boat rides which may significantly aggravate previous back conditions.
- Once in the water, there is normally no strain on the back but if positively buoyant it may necessitate swimming with the back and neck hyperextended to keep the fins high and thrusting downwards.
- Paraesthesia and numbness of the legs, a common complication of pre-existing lumbar spondylosis and PID, may be confused with symptoms of decompression illness (DCI).

Consider the risk of aggravating low back pain from a pre-existing back condition (a proven, regular and minor risk).

**This risk may be reduced using correct lifting techniques and getting assistance especially whilst kitting up.**

Consider the risk of confusing paraesthesia and numbness of the lower limbs from a pre-existing back condition with symptoms of DCI (a possible, remote and moderate risk).

**This risk may be reduced by limiting the depth and frequency of dives, always ascending slowly and having a safety stop before surfacing.**

Consider the analgesic medications being taken.

## FRACTURES

Common e.g., broken arm or leg

- Any fracture will disrupt and limit mobility and agility.
- It has been suggested that an injured area, e.g., a fracture site, may have altered gas uptake/ elimination and be more vulnerable to bubble formation and possible localised decompression illness. However, this has never been proven experimentally or clinically.

Consider the risk of reduced mobility and agility.

**This risk may be reduced by delaying diving until full function and strength are restored.**

Consider the risk of an increased incidence of decompression illness (a possible, rare and moderate risk).

**This risk may be reduced by limiting the depth and frequency of dives, always ascending slowly and incorporating a safety stop before surfacing.**

**We recommend that diving is delayed for a period which approximates twice the time for union which, as a rule of thumb, is twice the length of time in a plaster cast.**

## LUMBAR LAMINECTOMY

Spinal fusion

- Surgery to the lumbar spine frequently indicates a history of severe and chronic back pain. The diver may be taking long-term narcotic analgesic medication.
- There is often loss of mobility, ongoing back pain and neurological symptoms and signs such as numbness and muscle weakness.
- The disruption of the paravertebral venous plexus during such surgery has been suggested to predispose to spinal decompression illness but there is no evidence of this effect.

Consider the risk of aggrravating low back pain and its complications.

**This risk may be reduced using correct lifting techniques and getting assistance especially whilst kitting up.**

Consider the risk of narcotic medication.

Consider the risk of an increased incidence of spinal decompression illness (a possible, rare and moderate risk).

**This risk may be reduced by limiting the depth and frequency of dives, always ascending slowly and incorporating a safety stop before surfacing.**

## LATERAL EPICONDYLITIS

Tennis elbow, Tank carrier's elbow

- Carrying scuba tanks by grasping the valve stem and lifting vertically (which involves wrist pronation with dorsiflexion) can cause or aggravate this condition (Barr).

Consider the risk of aggravating pre-existing lateral epicondylitis.

**This risk may be reduced by avoiding carrying scuba tanks by their valve. Special tank carry slings have been designed.**

## ORTHOPAEDIC PINS AND PLATES, JOINT PROSTHESES

- The underlying condition necessitating the surgery needs to be determined and assessed.
- The function, mobility and stability of the affected area need to be assessed e.g., hip prostheses are susceptible to dislocation by excessive abduction. This could occur manoeuvring underwater, slipping on a wet deck, and clambering over the side of an inflatable dingy.
- In the case of metallic joint replacements, divers often notice a change in their buoyancy characteristics; they may need to adjust their weighting due to their newly acquired internal weights – the artificial joints. If one hip or knee is replaced, the diver may also tend to tilt or rotate to that side and may need to redistribute their weights to offset this.
- There is no evidence to suggest that metal, polymers, ceramics and composite materials within the body are a focus for bubble formation or predispose to decompression illness.
- Divers with hip replacements need to be careful in avoiding excessive abduction which can predispose to dislocation.
- If any orthopaedic hardware protrudes from the skin e.g., K wires, immersion would greatly increase the risk of infection.

Consider the risks of the underlying pathology requiring orthopaedic surgery.

Consider the risk of the stability of the replaced joint.

Consider the risk of infection.

**We would not recommend any diving if the integrity of the skin is compromised.**

## PECTUS EXCAVATUM

Funnel chest

- The depression of the body of the sternum and xiphoid process combined with the inward curving of the costal cartilages and adjacent ribs can predispose to repeated respiratory infections, decreased stamina and endurance and chest pain.
- If severe, it can be surgically corrected when vital capacity can be increased by a mean of 11% (Fonkalsrud).
- Surgical repair consists of subperiosteal resection of abnormal cartilage, transverse wedge osteotomy of the anterior sternum and internal support with a steel strut for 6 months. This procedure does not enter the pleural space.

Consider the risk of diminished vital capacity reducing endurance.

- This risk may be reduced by checking the vital capacity specifically and, if greatly reduced, having the diver's fitness fully assessed in the pool.

## PNEUMOCYSTS

- An air-containing cyst in bones is extremely rare but would be subject to barotrauma.
- It is usually asymptomatic and the diver would be unaware of its presence. Two cases of pneumocysts causing pain whilst diving have been reported (Robinet) and a third in the iliac crest has been documented by one of the authors (Azzopardi, personal communication).

Consider the risk of barotrauma causing pain in the region of the pneumocyst whilst diving.

**Any diver with a pneumocyst should seek specialist treatment before diving.**

## TEMPOROMANDIBULAR DISORDERS AND MYOFACIAL PAIN

e.g., Temporo-mandibular Joint Dysfunction Syndrome (TMJDS)

- This is a complex group of disorders. Anyone with the disorder should be warned that anxiety in divers is often associated with biting hard on the regulator mouthpiece aggravating pain in the temporomandibular joint (TMJ) or the muscles of the face, especially the muscles of mastication (Pinto).
- Some divers presenting with ear pain suggestive of otitis externa, yet with no sign of the infection were noted to have their regulator hose coming around the same side as their pain, which might create unbalanced stress on the TM joints (Muth).
- Most commercially available regulator mouthpieces have interdental bite blocks between the canine and premolar teeth. The lack of posterior support could cause abnormal loads on the myofacial muscles and TMJ (Hobson).

Consider the risk of diving aggravating a pre-existing TMJDS.

**This risk may be reduced by warning the diver of the problem and advising them to relax their mouthpiece grip whilst diving and even reduce their dive durations.**

Some divers get relief by using a custom-made regulator mouthpiece incorporating posterior dental support and ensuring the interocclusal rest space is not exceeded.

## SCOLIOSIS

- Decreased vital capacity may occur in people with severe thoracic curves (>60°), especially in the presence of thoracic lordosis. This will not cause any air trapping but could reduce exercise tolerance.

- Certain surgical procedures e.g., anterior fusions and thoracoplasties may cause pleural adhesions.

Consider the risk of restricted lung function reducing exercise tolerance.

Consider the risk of post-operative pleural adhesions.

## FURTHER READING:


1. Barr L L, Martin L R. Tank carrier's lateral epicondylitis: Case reports and a new cause for an old entity. SPUMS J 1991; 21(1): 35-37
2. Barr L L, Brunt D, Martin LR. Tank carrier's lateral epicondylitis: A biomechanical rationale for injury and prevention. SPUMS J 1991; 21(1): 37-41
3. Bradford D S, Tay B K, Hu S S. Adult scoliosis: surgical indications, operative management, complications and outcomes. Spine 1999; 24(24): 2617-29
4. Cush C. The straight scoop on spinal care for scuba divers. Alert Diver Mar/Apr 1996: 31-3
5. Hobson R S, Newton J P. Dental evaluation of scuba diving mouthpieces using a subject assessment index and radiological analysis of jaw position. Br J Sports Med 2001; 35: 84-8
6. Fonkalsrud E W, Dunn J C, Atkinson J B. Repair of excavatum deformities: 30 years of experience with 375 patients. Ann Surg 2000; 231(3): 443-8
7. Grant S M, Johnson F. Diver's mouth syndrome: a report of two cases and construction of custom-made regulator mouthpieces. Dent Update 1998; 25(6): 254-6
8. Hobson R S. Airway efficiency during the use of scuba diving mouthpieces. 1996; Br J Sports Med; 30(2): 145-147
9. Hopkirk J R, Pullan M J, Fraser J R. Pleurodesis: The results of treatment for spontaneous pneumothorax in the Royal Air Force. Av Sp Env Med 1983; 54(2): 158-60
10. Muth C M, Delb W, Iro H. HBO Centre, Homburg/Saar. ENT-Dept., University of Saarland, D-66424 Homburg/Saar, Germany. Newton J P, Hobson R S, Sturrock K C. The design and construction of customised mouthpieces for subaqua diving. Eur J Prosthodont Restor Dent 1995; 3(5): 223-226
11. Pinto O F. Temporomandibular joint problems in underwater activities. J Pros Dent 1966; 16: 772-81 Robinet C, Guillou L, Colineau X, Paoletti H, Pujol A, Muyard B, Solacroup J C. Intraosseous Pneumatocysts of the ileum on a diver. Bulleti de Medecine Subaquatique et Hyperbare 1997; 7(2): 33-41
12. Meucci R, Fassa A, Faria NMX. Prevalence of chronic low back pain: Systematic review. Revista de Saude Publica. Oct 201549:1-10. doi:10.1590/S0034-8910.2015049005874
13. Taddy J J. Scuba diving and TMD. Cranio 1993; 11(1): 73-4
14. Upadhyay S S, Mullaji A B, Luk K D, Leong J C. Relation of spinal and thoracic cage deformities and their flexibilities with altered pulmonary functions in adolescent idiopathic scoliosis. Spine 1995; 20: 2415-20

# Neurological Diseases

# 18

## POINTS TO PONDER

- Diving demands full consciousness, coordinated movements and normal muscle power. Any loss or clouding of consciousness whilst diving may quickly result in drowning.
- Uncontrolled descent with no ear equalization may initially result in severe aural barotrauma and ultimately pulmonary barotrauma. Uncontrolled ascent may quickly result in pulmonary barotrauma and cerebral arterial gas embolism (AGE).
- Decompression illness (DCI) frequently presents with varying neurological symptoms, e.g., paraesthesia, numbness, and weakness. In any diver who has a medical condition that may also present with such symptoms, there is a risk that any symptom appearing, even days after a dive, may be ignored with the risk that DCI is undertreated. Alternatively, the symptom may be misdiagnosed as DCI leading to overtreatment.
- The brain and spinal cord are susceptible to decompression illness (DCI) because myelin is a lipid with a high affinity for nitrogen. The spinal cord is especially susceptible to DCI (Bond).

## ATTENTION DEFICIT / HYPERACTIVITY DISEASE (ADHD)

Attention deficit disability (ADD), neurodevelopment disorders

- Although traditionally characterized as a disorder of childhood (with a prevalence of 4-8%) (Faraone), two-thirds of cases progress into adulthood.
- Common features include attention problems, hyperreactivity, impulsiveness and mood swings.
- It is commonly associated with anxiety disorders and substance abuse.
- The risk of seizures is increased up to threefold.
- Psychostimulant medications, mexamphetamine and methylphenidate (Ritalin) are first-line treatments. Paradoxically the psychostimulant medication can improve attention and focus and create a possible danger of 'over-concentration and over-focus' where awareness of the outer world is compromised.

Consider the risk of inattention, hyperactivity and impulsiveness.

**This risk can be minimized by waiting until the diver is 18 years old and shows only mild symptoms.**

Consider the risk of psychostimulant medication.

**This risk can be minimized by only permitting divers controlled with one medication, who have no side effects and are fully compliant.**

These recommendations only apply to divers wanting open water certification so they may dive independently. Many dive companies run 'adaptive' dive training courses and dives for physically and mentally handicapped divers with specially trained instructors and assistants and greater diver support. It may be possible for other ADHD sufferers to enjoy the possibilities of diving in this specialized environment.

## AUTISM SPECTRUM DISORDER (ASD)

Autism Disorder, Asperger's Syndrome, Pervasive Development Disorder

- ASD is a complex developmental condition that involves persistent challenges in social interaction, speech and nonverbal communication, and restricted/repetitive and unusual sensory–motor behaviours. It is now seen as a spectrum that can range from very mild to severe.
- It is commonly diagnosed by 3 years of age but diagnosis can be delayed until adulthood. It is a life-long condition.
- Although 'high-functioning autism' is not an official medical term it is used to describe people with ASD who can speak, read, write, and handle basic life skills like eating and getting dressed and can often live independently. However even they have a hard time with social interaction and communication. They are very devoted to routine and order and might have repetitive and restrictive habits.
- Researchers at Midwestern University surveyed a group of kids and young adults with autism spectrum disorders and their response to scuba diving. The study found that four major themes emerged: feeling better about myself and what I can do, finding sensory freedom in the water, social participation, and not being defined by disability or "everybody is equal underwater".

Consider the risks of breaking routines and stretching comfort zones increasing anxiety in an underwater environment,

Consider the risks of poor communication and understanding whilst training.

Consider the risks of poor social interaction and communication with fellow divers.

Consider the risks of anxiety caused by under and over-sensory stimulation.

**We would not recommend anyone with ASD to train to scuba dive in a regular training course. High-functioning autistic persons could follow 'adaptive training' courses with specialized courses for disabled divers where timelines, teaching methods, supervision and diving plans are all tailored to the needs of the diver.**

## BELL'S PALSY

- This presumed viral neuropathy causes unilateral facial weakness and pain. Although usually transient the weakness can remain permanently and cause difficulty in retaining a regulator in the mouth.
- The main complication is exposure keratitis from an inadequately protected cornea. A similar presentation can occur from facial baroparesis after diving.

Consider the risk of the regulator being easily dislodged.

Consider the risk of exposure keratitis from seawater irritation whilst diving.

**This risk may be reduced by ensuring the eye fully closes when blinking.**

**We would not recommend diving until there was a full resolution of the pain and weakness. Should a residual weakness occur, it should be certain that the diver can firmly retain the regulator mouthpiece and that the eye closes completely while blinking.**

## CHRONIC FATIGUE SYNDROME / MYALGIC ENCEPHALOPATHY (ME)

- Characteristic features include chronic persisting or relapsing fatigue of a generalized nature, exacerbated by minor exercise.
- There is frequent impairment of concentration, short-term memory loss and cognitive difficulties.

Consider the risk of easy fatigue reducing exercise tolerance.

Consider the risk of poor concentration and cognition reducing the mental ability to dive safely.

**We would discourage anyone with chronic fatigue to dive but if highly motivated to attend a special course with added supervision and a more relaxed schedule, we would allow diving in this context.**

## DEGENERATIVE NERVOUS SYSTEM DISORDERS

e.g., Dementia, Motor Neuron Disease, Parkinson's Disease

- These conditions decrease mental alertness, concentration, coordination and cognition.
- They begin insidiously and run a gradual progressive course. Often by the time the diagnosis is made, there will be significant disabling symptoms but with greater awareness and diagnostic acumen, early diagnosis is becoming more common.

Consider the risk of an increased incidence of decompression illness (DCI) (a possible, remote and moderate risk).

Consider the risk of reduced concentration, coordination and cognition (a plausible, regular and major risk).

**We would not recommend anyone with any detectable dementia to dive.**

## EPILEPSY

- Any loss of consciousness or awareness underwater will increase the risk of drowning.
- There is also a significant risk of pulmonary barotrauma and cerebral arterial gas embolism if a diver is brought up to the surface whilst convulsing and not breathing regularly.
- Underwater, a diver may be exposed to many possible triggering stimuli for convulsions including glare, flickering light, sensory deprivation, hyperventilation, anxiety and cold water. Alcohol and sleep deprivation may also lower the threshold for a convulsion. If a person is on anticonvulsant medication, their suppressed seizure focus may be activated by such conditions.
- Even after cessation of anticonvulsant medication, there is a real risk of recurrence. In one study that followed epileptics for over 30 years over one-third suffered a relapse after stopping the medication. Two-thirds of the relapses occurred within three years but some happened after much longer periods (Sillanpää). Several 'near-miss' diving accidents have been reported in divers after several seizure-free years (Smart).
- Many convulsions in early childhood are not considered to be a risk factor in later life. These include neonatal convulsions with no subsequent neurological problems, simple febrile convulsions, convulsions secondary to breath-holding attacks, drug ingestion and sepsis or meningitis, where there are no subsequent neurological complications.
- Recent advancements in brain imaging and neurosurgery are curing previously uncontrolled epilepsy.

Consider the risk of convulsing underwater (a proven, remote and major risk).

**The risk may be reduced if the EEG is normal, there are no structural brain lesions and diving is delayed for at**

**least a five-year, convulsion-free period whilst off medication. After curative surgery, a five-year convulsion-free period is also advised.**

Consider the risk of any anticonvulsant medication.

**The South Pacific Underwater Medical Society recommends that "a candidate with a history of fits (apart from febrile convulsions), or unexplained blackouts should be strongly advised against diving. Any condition associated with fits or blackouts will be a grave risk to life during diving."**

**The United Kingdom Sport Diving Medical Committee (UKSDMC) is less stringent - "an epileptic is permitted to dive after five years free from fits and off medication. Where the fits were exclusively nocturnal, this can be reduced to three years."**

**We would not recommend anyone with a history of epilepsy who is on medication to dive.**

**We would discourage anyone with a history of epilepsy who has been off medication and convulsion-free for a minimum of five years to dive. If they are determined to continue and have a normal EEG and there are no structural brain lesions, we would highlight the risks and advise them to avoid any preventable aggravating factors, e.g., alcohol, sleep deprivation and hyperventilation. We would advise that their buddy is fully informed of their past condition.**

## HEADACHES

- A severe headache can be disabling if occurring during a dive. It is important to determine the aetiology of headaches of divers who suffer from them frequently.
    - » Benign Exertional Headaches can be caused by vigorous exercise, e.g., swimming. They typically are pulsating global headaches that last about 5 minutes but may persist for hours as a steady dull global headache.
    - » Carbon Dioxide Retention Headaches can be caused by nocturnal hypoventilation due to obstructive sleep apnoea, periodic breathing or neuromuscular respiratory weakness and frequently cause morning headaches. They can be aggravated in divers who "skip breathe" (i.e., slow down their respiratory rate or intermittently hold their breath to conserve air or control buoyancy). Less common causes are restrictive wetsuit or buoyancy compensators,closed or semi-closed rebreathing apparatus and heavy exercise. The headache typically is throbbing and appears slowly, is bitemporal, bifrontal or bi-occipital and lasts 10-30 minutes. It is typically associated with mental confusion and dizziness.
    - » Ice cream headaches occur within seconds of eating or drinking something cold. Pain typically lasts 20-30 seconds but can persist for up to 5 minutes. It is thought to be a reflex response triggered by stimulation of the trigeminal nerve. If the diver is very sensitive the headache may be caused by jumping into cold water and may be avoided by wearing a neoprene hood.
    - » Migraine. See the section on migraine
    - » Sinusitis. Chronic sinusitis can often present as recurrent headaches. See the section on Sinusitis.
    - » Temporomandibular Joint Dysfunction (TMJD). See section TMJD
    - » Tension Headaches are probably the commonest cause of daily headaches. It is commonly bilateral and described as a band-like sensation around the head. There may be an excessive contraction of the jaw and facial muscles. They can be aggravated by mask straps being fitted too tightly (goggle headache) (Jacobsen). Treatment may include tricyclic antidepressants.

» Trigeminal neuralgia is a severe stabbing pain more commonly affecting the second and third divisions of the trigeminal nerve. Trigger areas are often in the nasolabial groove aggravated by the mask. Treatment may include anti-convulsant drugs.

## HEAD INJURY

Fractured skull, Unconsciousness, Post-traumatic amnesia, Sub-dural hematoma

- Head injuries are associated with brain injury. Even after only momentary unconsciousness or amnesia, there can be brain damage. The pathology may include contusion, hematoma and diffuse axonal injury.
- The main risks are whether any residual neurological damage may diminish cognition or provoke post-traumatic convulsions.
- The severity of the head injury can be related to post-traumatic amnesia (PTA), defined as the time from the head injury to the laying down of continuous memory, with <30mins = mild, 30mins –24hrs = moderate, and >24hrs = severe.
- Other complications, which may indicate a severe head injury, may include intracranial haemorrhage e.g., subdural hematoma, depressed skull fracture, penetrating head injury, rhinorrhoea or otorrhea longer than 7 days, convulsions at the time of head injury and post-traumatic meningitis or encephalitis.
- Post-traumatic epilepsy is more likely after severe head injuries. Sixty per cent will present in the first year, 24% in 1-4 years and 16% after 4 years. Only about 1% of uncomplicated mild head injuries will have a convulsion.
- A post-concussion syndrome can cause recurring headaches, dizziness, poor concentration and memory, unsteadiness and irritability. It can be accompanied by anxiety, depression and personality changes.
- Damaged brain tissue may be more susceptible to decompression illness (DCI).

Consider the risk of a post-traumatic neurological deficit diminishing memory and understanding, reducing the diver's ability to dive safely (a possible, remote and moderate risk).

**This risk may be reduced by having the deficit functionally assessed in its relevance to diving.**

Consider the risk of a convulsion occurring during a dive (a possible, rare and major risk).

**This risk may be reduced by delaying diving after a head injury. Suggested delays are at least three years following an uncomplicated severe head injury, a year following a moderate head injury and a month after a mild head injury.**

Consider the risk of increased incidence of DCI in anyone with a residual neurological deficit (a possible, remote and moderate risk).

**This risk may be reduced by limiting the depth and frequency of diving and always incorporating a safety stop.**

**After a severe head injury, we do not recommend any further diving.**

**After a moderate head injury, we recommend a delay of one year. Even after a mild head injury, we recommend a delay of a month.**

**We explain the risks to the prospective diver and we would recommend that no one with a history of head injury with amnesia, loss of consciousness or convulsions continue diving.**

# INTRACRANIAL HAEMORRHAGE

Subarachnoid haemorrhage

- Such a bleed reflects a structural change in the cerebral circulation, usually an aneurysm, rarely an A-V malformation. This needs to be determined and assessed.
- There is a recurrent rate of haemorrhages of 2% per annum.

Consider the risk of a recurrent bleed being aggravated whilst diving (a possible, rare and major risk).

Consider the risk of a convulsion occurring whilst diving (a possible, rare and major risk).

**This risk may be reduced by delaying diving for five years.**

**If the aneurysm had been successfully surgically clipped, there was no other structural abnormality of the cerebral circulation or neurological deficit and there had been no convulsions we would recommend diving after five years.**

## Cerebral Vascular Accident (CVA)

- This intracerebral haemorrhage or infarction is usually caused by cerebral artery disease or emboli. Other causes include bleeding disorders and arteritis.
- There is often a high risk of recurrent bleeds. After a stroke, there is a 5% per year chance of another stroke and a 5% per year chance of a myocardial infarction.
- Convulsions can commence after such cerebral insults.
- Residual neurological deficits are common and often severe, e.g., hemiplegia, but can be unobtrusive yet very disabling.

Consider the risk of a neurological deficit affecting performance during a dive.

**This risk may be reduced by having the deficit functionally assessed for its relevance to diving.**

Consider the risk of convulsions occurring during a dive (a possible, rare and major risk).

Consider the risk of increased incidence of DCI in anyone with a residual neurological deficit (a possible, remote and moderate risk).

**This risk may be reduced by limiting the depth and frequency of diving and always ascending slowly and doing a safety stop.**

Consider the risk of co-existing coronary artery disease.

**This risk may be reduced by a full cardiovascular assessment before diving.**

**We would not usually recommend anyone with a history of CVA to dive. If the cause was fully reversible e.g., drug-induced thrombocytopenia, then we would obtain a specialist neurological assessment to assess neurological function and confirm adequate function before recommending diving. A delay of at least five years after the CVA will reduce the likelihood of a convulsion.**

# INTRACRANIAL SURGERY

- The underlying pathology of the surgery needs to be determined and assessed.
- Many patients are left with post-operative residual neurological deficits.

- Any intracranial surgery must leave scar tissue on the brain. This could be a focus for seizure activity.
- Damaged brain tissue may be more susceptible to decompression illness (DCI).
- Defects of the skull may need special protection from physical trauma underwater.
- Surgery to the pituitary gland requiring an intranasal approach would leave a bony defect in the sphenoidal sinus wall, which may be more prone to sinus barotrauma leading to a pneumocephalus.

Consider the risk of the underlying pathology.

Consider the risk of any residual neurological deficit affecting performance underwater.

Consider the risk of convulsions occurring whilst diving (a possible, rare and major risk).

Consider the risk of increased incidence of DCI (a possible, rare and moderate risk)

**This risk may be reduced by limiting the time and frequency of diving and always ascending slowly and doing a safety stop.**

**We would recommend diving only after uncomplicated surgery for a benign condition with no history of post-operative convulsions or neurological deficit.**

**We would still recommend a five-year delay before diving.**

**We would not recommend anyone with a history of complex cranial surgery involving parenchymal manipulation, and/or a history of convulsions, to dive.**

## MIGRAINE

- Sudden attacks of migraine can produce disabling symptoms such as severe headache, vomiting, vertigo, severe muscular weakness and clouding of consciousness.
- Occasionally migraine can be aggravated by anxiety, travel, exercise, swimming, cold or even scuba diving itself. It has been suggested that both cerebral venous bubbles and carbon dioxide retention may both aggravate a migraine by inducing vasodilation. Hypercapnia is a recognized trigger for cluster headaches (Hannerz).
- An association has been reported between migraine with aura and the presence of right to left shunts detected with transcranial doppler. Divers who suffered neurological DCI and who had large patent foramen ovale (PFO) were noted to have a high incidence of migraine with aura. Their migraines were also noted to diminish after surgical correction of the PFO (Wilmshurst).
- Some symptoms of migraine can be confused with those of decompression illness (DCI). These include paraesthesia, tiredness, muscular weakness, headache, dizziness and nausea.
- Ergot derivatives, e.g., ergotamine and methysergide can cause pleuritis and pleural fibrosis as late as 2 years after initiation of therapy.

Consider the risk of disabling symptoms occurring whilst diving (a plausible, remote and moderate risk).

Consider the risk of migraine symptoms being confused with DCI after a dive (a plausible, remote and moderate risk).

**This risk may be reduced by limiting depths and frequency of dives and always ascending slowly and incorporating a safety stop.**

Consider the risk of diving aggravating a migraine (a plausible, rare and moderate risk).

Consider the risk that migraine with aura may be a sign of a large intracardiac right to left shunt which may predispose to serious neurological DCI (a possible, rare and major risk).

**This risk may be reduced by having transthoracic contrast echocardiography to exclude an intracardiac right to left shunt.**

Consider the risk of side effects of prophylaxis medication.

**We would not recommend anyone with frequent disabling migraines or migraines with auras to dive.**

**We advise all migraine sufferers not to dive if they have had a migraine in the previous 24 hours and to avoid any aggravating factors. We also advise them of the possible confusion of their migraine symptoms with DCI and the possible need for recompression should this occur.**

**If diving aggravates migraine, then diving should cease.**

## MUSCULAR DYSTROPHY

Duchenne Muscular Dystrophy, Becker Muscular Dystrophy, Erb's Adult Muscular Dystrophy, Limb-Girdle Muscle Dystrophy, Myotonic Dystrophy

- These progressive hereditary degenerative diseases of skeletal muscle usually afflict children who are severely handicapped by adolescence.
- Those forms with a later onset will have significant muscular weakness and atrophy.
- Myotonia, the prolonged contraction of certain muscles, especially the hands and tongue, may be a feature of the disease.

Consider the risk of muscular weakness affecting the diver's ability to enter and exit the water, swim independently and perform a rescue.

**This risk may be reduced by limiting diving to disabled level 2 or 3.**

Consider the risk of increased incidence of decompression illness (DCI).

**The risk may be reduced by limiting the depth and frequency of diving and always incorporating a safety stop.**

**We would not normally recommend anyone with this condition to dive.**

## MYASTHENIA GRAVIS

- This disease is characterized by fluctuant weakness of certain voluntary muscles. It may be insidious in onset and present as exertional stridor. Repeated or persistent activity of a muscle group exhausts its contracting power leading to progressive weakness. It usually occurs in young adults.
- Spontaneous remission may occur but is usually short-lived and it continues a slow progression unless treated.
- Medication with anticholinesterases may cause nausea and vomiting, and increases salivation and bronchial secretions. Muscle cramps and weakness can also occur.

Consider the risk of muscular weakness affecting the diver's ability to enter and exit the water, swim independently and perform a rescue.

**This risk may be reduced if the diver restricts diving to disabled level 2 or 3.**

**The risk will be dependent on the amount of weakness and exercise capacity. We would discourage anyone with the condition to dive.**

## MULTIPLE SCLEROSIS (MS)

- This common demyelinating disease tends to attack young people. The diagnosis may be uncertain at the onset and awaits the development of more characteristic symptoms and signs.
- Initial manifestations are often optic neuritis, ataxia, nystagmus and brainstem signs, such as diplopia, vertigo and vomiting. Other symptoms include weakness, paraesthesia, impaired vision, dysarthria, intention tremor, impairment of deep sensation, paraparesis, and alteration in emotional response.
- The most common sign is fatigue.
- About 50% of people with MS present as an intermittently progressive disease. A relapse is not a sudden event but comes on over hours or days.
- The susceptibility of demyelinated nervous tissue to decompression illness (DCI) is not known.
- The symptoms of MS may mimic decompression illness (DCI) (Jan).
- Any such symptom, which occurs within days of a dive, must be assumed to be DCI and treated as such.

Consider the risk of muscular weakness affecting the diver's ability to enter and exit the water, swim independently and perform a rescue.

**This risk may be reduced by limiting diving to disability level 2 or 3.**

Consider the risk of symptoms of MS being confused with DCI requiring recompression.

**This risk may be reduced by limiting the depth and frequency of dives and always ascending slowly and incorporating a safety stop.**

There are rare anecdotal reports of people with a history of optic neuritis becoming blind when given hyperbaric oxygen (HBO) treatment, even if it was not active at the time. This may be relevant to recreational diving if hyperbaric treatment is required e.g., treatment of decompression illness.

**We recommend anyone who is symptom-free and in remission to dive but emphasize the warning about symptom confusion with DCI.**

## VENTRICULOPERITONEAL/ATRIAL SHUNTS

- These are usually inserted for hydrocephalus due to congenital abnormalities or post-natal causes such as meningitis, intracranial haemorrhage or tumour. There may be residual brain damage depending on the cause of the original obstruction and the speed at which the hydrocephalus was relieved.
- Shunt malfunctions commonly present as convulsions. There may be a history of convulsions from the underlying cause of the hydrocephalus.
- Low-grade infection often prevents the valves from being permanently effective and requires frequent shunt revision.
- The occipital burr hole approach has a higher incidence of epilepsy (even after only one pass of the cannula) than the parietal burr hole approach. Fourth ventricular shunts also have more complications.
- There is a concern that an atrial shunt could aggravate bubble formation in supersaturated blood.
- As the shunt system and the valve mechanism are filled with cerebral spinal fluid (CSF), it will be subjected to the same pressure changes as the ventricles, atria and peritoneum.
- One make of shunt has been dry-tested to 4 ATA and found to perform normally (Huang).

Consider the risk of convulsions whilst diving from a malfunction or infection of the shunt (a possible, remote and major risk).

**This risk may be reduced if there is no history of convulsion or any infection of a long-standing shunt.**

Consider the risk of decompression illness being aggravated by an atrial shunt (a possible, remote and moderate risk).

**This risk may be reduced by limiting the depth and frequency of diving and always incorporating a safety stop to avoid bubble formation and minimize nitrogen loads.**

**We would not usually recommend anyone with this condition to dive.**

## FURTHER READING:


1. Abul MM, Alam K, O'Driscoll K, Murphy P S. Acute inspiratory stridor: a presentation of myasthenia gravis. J Laryngol Otol 1999; 113(12): 1114-5

2. Bond J P, Kirschner D A. Spinal cord myelin is vulnerable to decompression. Mol Chem Neuropathol 1997; 30(3): 273-88

3. Cheshire W P Jr, Ott M C. Headache in Divers. Headache 2001; 41: 235-47

4. Do Rosario MG, Bell SG, Sander JW. Epilepsy and recreational scuba diving: an absolute contraindication or can there be exceptions? A call for discussion. Epilepsia 2007 May;48(5):851-8. doi: 10.1111/j.1528-1167.2007.01045.x. MID: 17508997 DOI: 10.1111/j.1528-1167.2007.01045.x

5. Dreifus F E. Epileptics and scuba diving. JAMA 1985; 253(13): 1877-8

6. Francis J. Mechanisms of Spinal Cord Injury in Decompression Illness. SPUMS J 1998; 28(1): 29-41

7. Friedberg F, Dechene L, McKenzie M J 2nd, Fontanette R. Symptom patterns in long-duration chronic fatigue syndrome. J Psychosom Res 2000; 48(1): 59-68

8. Green R D, Keitch D R. Head Injury and diving: a review. J R Nav Med Serv.1985 winter; 71(3):144-9 Greer H. CNS considerations in scuba diving. Alert Diver May/June 1999: 34-38

9. Jacobsen R I. More "goggle headache": supraorbital neuralgia (letter). N Engl J Med 1983. 308: 1363

10. Huang E T, Hardy K R, Stubbs J M, Lowe R A, Thom S R. Ventriculo-peritoneal shunt performance under hyperbaric conditions. Undersea Hyper Med 2000; 27(4): 191-4

11. Jan M H, Janosky C. Multiple sclerosis presenting as decompression illness. Undersea Hyper Med 2001; 28 (Supp): 48

12. Juul-Jensen P, Foldspan A. Natural history of epileptic seizures. 1983 Epilepsia; 24: 297-301

13. Juul-Jensen P. Frequency of recurrence of discontinuance of anticonvulsant therapy in patients with epileptic seizures. Epilepsia 1964; 5: 352-7

14. Hannerz J, Jogestrand T. Provocation of unilateral pain in cluster headache patients by breathing CO2. Headache 1995; 35: 38-43

15. Knappe UJ, Moskopp D, Gerlach R, Conrad J, Flitsch J, Honegger JB. Consensus on Postoperative Recommendations After Transsphenoidal Surgery. Exp Clin Endocrinol Diabetes 2019 Jan;127(1):29-36. doi: 10.1055/a-0664-7710. Epub 2018 Aug 21. PMID: 30130806 DOI: 10.1055/a-0664-7710

16. Lee M, Leahu D, Weiner H L, Abbott R, Wisoff J H, Epstein F J. Complications of fourth-ventricular shunts. Paed Neurosurg 1995; 22(6): 309-13

17. Naradzay J F, Brown B J, Rolnick M A, Doherty R J. Cerebral ventricular Shunts. J Emerg Med 1999; 17(2): 311-22

18. Pedley T A. Discontinuation of antiepileptic drugs. New Eng J Med 1988; 318: 982-6

19. Sillanpää M, Schmidt D. Prognosis of seizure recurrence after stopping antiepileptic drugs in seizure-free patients: A

long-term population-based study of childhood-onset epilepsy. Epilepsy Behav. 2006;8:713-9

20. Smart D, Lippman J. Epilepsy, scuba diving and risk assessment. Near misses and the need for ongoing vigilance. Diving Hyperb Med 2013 Mar;43(1):37-41. PMID: 23508661

21. Vajda F J E, Antiepileptic drug withdrawal: can the response be predicted? Current Therapeutics. 1994; 35 : 17-21
Salazar C, De Saa M, Aparicio M, Garcia B, Casadol. Myasthenia gravis: Otorhinolaryngological considerations. Acta Otorrinolaringol Esp 2000; 51(1): 92-6

22. Wilmshurst P T, Nightingale S, Walsh K P, Morrison W L. Effect on migraine of closure of cardiac right-to-left shunts to prevent recurrence of decompression illness or stroke or for hemodynamic reasons. Lancet 2000; 356: 1648-51

# Ophthalmic Issues 19

## POINTS TO PONDER

- Whilst diving the diver should be able to enjoy the visual beauty of the underwater environment. Without a mask, the diver's vision would be approximately -40 dioptres and everything is severely blurred. The mask restores the air/cornea interface and eliminates the induced hypermetropia.
- The diver should also be able:
    - » to read gauges showing air pressure, depth, dive time and decompression requirements, as well as read a compass.
    - » to locate and navigate entry and exit points.
    - » to locate and recognize their buddy.
- The eyeball is fluid-filled and attains ambient pressure with no volume change.
- Mask squeeze can subject the eyeball and skin within the mask to considerable pressure, sufficient to cause multiple skin petechiae and subconjunctival haemorrhage. In extreme cases, it can cause hyphaema and subperiosteal orbital haemorrhage.
- The diving mask reduces the sideward range of vision from 180° to about 80°. It also reduces the vertical range of vision which makes visual checks of equipment worn on the body difficult.
- The refraction of light at the water/air interface at the mask causes the apparent size of objects to be magnified by one-third and their distance to be reduced by one-quarter.
- As light travels through water it is attenuated by absorption and scattering. It becomes darker with increasing depth. Even in clear water only about 20% of incident light reaches 10m (33ft) and 1% reaches 85 m (260 ft). In dirty water, this is reduced further.
- As light passes through water, different wavelengths are selectively absorbed. Red colours disappear by 10m (33 ft) and yellow colours by 23m (75 ft). By 30m (100 ft), only blues and greens remain. Artificial light from torches and camera flashes will re-introduce the full-colour range.

## CATARACT SURGERY

- Cataract surgery is now very common. The cataract is removed by phacoemulsification and an intraocular lens is inserted through a tiny incision of 2-3mm, which normally does not need sutures and has an inherent strength even before healing occurs.
- External healing of the wound normally only takes a few days, during which time diving should be avoided to reduce the risk of infection.

Consider the risk of wound infection.

**The risk can be reduced by waiting 1-2 months after surgery before diving.**

## CONJUNCTIVAL-DACRYOCYSTORHINOSTOMY

Jone's Tubes

- This repair of plugged nasolacrimal ducts creates a patent opening into the nose from the lacrimal caruncle. This will allow any water within the mask easy access into the nasal passages causing instant irritation.
- In reverse, it will allow air to travel up the lacrimal duct during a forced Valsalva manoeuvre and exit at the lacrimal punctum opening.

## COLOUR BLINDNESS

- Normal colour vision is not necessary forrecreational diving but is a compulsory requirement in professional commercial diving.

## CONTACT LENSES

- Both soft and hard lenses are used widely to correct both myopia and hyperopia. They are both worn extensively by people swimming, snorkelling and diving.
- Soft hydrogel lenses have a larger diameter (about 14 mm) and are less likely to be lost or washed out of the eye than the smaller hard lens (9 mm).
- Refractive errors greater than this range and certain conditions such as keratoconus, corneal scars and grafts demand the use of hard lenses.
- The original polymethylmethacrylate (PMMA) has been replaced by gas-permeable silicone or cellulose acetate lenses.
- Modern contact lenses are, for the purposes of recreational diving, all gas permeable.
- Extended-wear lenses, approved for up to 6-day continual usage and proposed 30-day continual usage, have a higher complication rate than daily-wear lenses. The complications are aggravated by the reduced oxygenation of the cornea as a result of the diminished tear flow. This can result in corneal oedema and infection, occasionally a devastating infection. Corneal ischaemia may be aggravated by diving.
- The main problem in using contact lenses is losing them while diving. If both lenses are lost by a diver with a severe bilateral refractory deficit they could be compromised for the rest of the dive. The cost of replacing a hard lens may be high.
- Contact with seawater may cause soft contact lenses to become tightly adherent to the cornea. The diver may experience recurrent mild ocular irritation and blurring of the vision after dives.

Consider the risk and cost of losing the lenses while diving.

**This risk may be reduced by wearing a prescription mask while diving. If contact lenses are worn, the mask should be firmly fitting with a good seal. If accidental flooding does occur, narrowing of the palpebral fissure may reduce the chance of the contact lens floating off until the mask has been cleared. When purposefully flooding, removing or replacing the mask close the eyes completely.**

- Consider the risk of corneal infection.

**This risk may be reduced by avoiding extended-wear lenses.**

**Soft disposable lenses are the most suitable for diving.**

**Extended-wear lenses are not recommended.**

## CORNEAL PATHOLOGY

- Corneal irregularities due to scarring or corneal dystrophy make the eye more susceptible to abrasions and ulceration. This will not normally affect the diver unless they are diving in contaminated water e.g., near sewerage outlets, when there is a danger of corneal infection.

## CORNEAL TRANSPLANT

- This usually involves a penetrating keratoplasty with a full-thickness, circumferential wound.
- Normally sutures will remain in place to strengthen the wound for up to a year.
- If the wound is subjected to a severe mask squeeze there is a danger of the wound opening.
- Onlay or lamellar grafts are sometimes used and being only partial thickness are inherently stable and resistant to infection once external healing has occurred.

Consider the risk of a severe mask squeeze reopening the wound (a possible, remote and major risk).

**This risk may be reduced by waiting 6-12 months in order for the wound to gain strength.**

## EXCIMER LASER KERATOTOMY

Photorefractive Keratotomy (PRK), Laser Assisted In-situ Keratomileusis (LASIK), Automated Lamellar Keratoplasty (ALK), Intrastromal Photorefractive Keratectomy (ISPK).

- These procedures have radically changed refractive surgery. The cornea can be resculptured without compromising its structural integrity and strength.
- Complications include transient overcorrection, excessive glare and halo affecting vision.

**There is no added risk associated with recreational scuba diving. Divers are recommended to wait two weeks post-operatively before diving.**

## GLAUCOMA

- A progressive visual loss due to a perfusion failure of the circulation of the anterior optic nerve. It is an ischemic disease. A common cause of ischemia is raised intraocular pressure.
- Diving raises both the intraocular and extraocular pressures. Saturation divers working at a depth of 240 m (800 ft) have an intraocular pressure of 19,000 mm Hg and work for weeks with no glaucoma, which depends not on the absolute pressure but the difference between the intraocular and extraocular pressures.
- Eye drops containing beta blockers are a common treatment for glaucoma. If these are absorbed systemically, they could provoke cardiac effects or bronchospasm or even reduce exercise tolerance.
- Oral carbonic anhydrase inhibitors, acetazolamide and methazolamide, are used when topical agents alone are insufficient or are not tolerated. As they affect carbon dioxide transport, they could enhance carbon dioxide retention which, when combined with exercise and depth, could aggravate carbon dioxide toxicity and enhance nitrogen narcosis and oxygen toxicity. They also can cause peripheral paraesthesia and electrolyte disturbances. Paraesthesia can be confused with decompression illness.
- Glaucoma filtering procedures e.g., trabeculectomy or sclerestomy involve producing a fistula to allow aqueous to drain

from the anterior chamber to the subconjunctival space. This closed system should be safe for diving but could be compromised if:

» a mask squeeze resulted in a subconjunctival haemorrhage and chemosis that compromised the function of the filter, or

» the conjunctival bleb was damaged and infection gained access to the anterior chamber resulting in endophthalmitis.

Consider the risk of complications of eye drops (a possible, remote and moderate risk).

**This risk may be reduced by punctate pressure after instilling the eye drops and ensuring that the diver has been on the medication for several weeks and has an appropriate cardiac response to exercise.**

Consider the risk of carbon dioxide retention when taking a carbonic anhydrase inhibitor (a possible, rare and moderate risk).

Consider the risk of trauma causing infection to the anterior chamber of the eye (a possible, rare and moderate risk).

**This risk may be reduced by avoiding mask squeeze by exhaling through the nose and protecting the face by always wearing the mask when in the water.**

## OPHTHALMIC SURGERY

- The structural integrity of the eyeball may be weakened and made more susceptible to rupture if exposed to direct trauma or severe mask squeeze.
- The eye may be more susceptible to serious infection, especially if diving postoperatively in contaminated water.
- During some surgical procedures, a tamponade of the vitreous cavity is created using air or gas into the eyeball which, when exposed to changes in pressure, could cause intraocular barotrauma causing intraocular haemorrhage.
- Before diving, it is important to check with the surgeon what convalescent period is recommended. Specific recommendations are given for the most significant procedures for divers in this text.

Consider the risk of infection.

**This risk may be reduced by waiting until the wound has fully healed.**

Consider the risk of intraocular barotrauma and retinal detachment.

**This risk may only be reduced by waiting until all gas in the eyeball has been resorbed.**

Consider the risk of rupture of the eyeball.

**This risk may be reduced by avoiding severe mask squeeze by exhaling through the nose and protecting the eyeball from direct blows by always keeping the facemask on the face.**

**Recommended minimum convalescent periods prior to diving after ophthalmic surgery have been given by Butler:**

| | | | |
|---|---|---|---|
| Penetrating keratoplasty | | | 6 months |
| Corneal laceration repair | | | 6 months |
| Cataract surgery | Non-corneal valve incision | | 3 months |
| | Corneal incision | Clear corneas | 2 months |
| | | Scleral tunnels | 1 month |
| Radial and astigmatic keratotomy | | | 3 months |
| Glaucoma filtering surgery | | | 2 months |
| Photorefractive surgery | | | 2 weeks |
| Pterygium surgery | | | 2 weeks |
| Conjunctival surgery | | | 2 weeks |
| Corneal suture removal | | | 1 week |
| Argon laser trabeculoplasty and Yag laser capsulotomy | | | No wait |
| Vitrectomy (no diving until all gas is fully resorbed) | | | 2 months |
| Retinal detachment repair | | | 2 months |
| Pneumatic retinopexy (no diving until all gas is fully resorbed) | | | 2 months |
| Sutured wound | | | 2 weeks |
| Skin grafting or granulating wound | | | Until epithelialization is complete |
| Enucleation | | | 2 weeks |
| Strabismus surgery | | | 2 weeks |

## ORBITAL IMPLANT

- A pressure-induced collapse of hollow silicone implants was reported in 3m (10 ft) of water. A hollow glass implant survived a test to 38m (115 ft).
- Modern orbital implants are porous and made from hydroxyapatite or polyethylene. They should be pressure resistant to recreational diving depths.

Consider the risk of collapse of the implant.

**Check the type of implant. We would not recommend diving whilst wearing any hollow implant.**

## PRESCRIPTION LENSES IN FACE MASKS

- Many dive shops and schools stock ready-made minus spherical form prescription lenses, ready for instant fitting into one or both eye apertures. There is no adjustment for astigmatism or individual distances between pupillary optical centres.
- Alternatively, an optician's prescription can be custom-made for the mask which corrects astigmatism and allows the exact interpupillary distance.
- Progressive lenses cannot be satisfactorily bonded to a dive mask. Divers with demands for critical near vision have been greatly facilitated by the development of lens design allowing 'free-form' lens surfacing to enhance bifocal vision, especially for presbyopia (Meister).

## RADIAL KERATOTOMY (RK), ASTIGMATIC KERATOTOMY (AK)

- These procedures involve several radial or curved cuts through 95% of the corneal thickness to the level of Descemet's membrane.
- RK is designed to increase the peripheral curvature of the cornea so the central area is flattened and corrects pre-existing myopia.
- AK is designed to correct the asymmetry or the cornea.
- In practice, the cuts often penetrate the full thickness of the cornea producing aqueous leaks and microscopic corneal perforations. This will weaken the cornea and make it susceptible to infection.
- Severe mask squeeze has the potential to move the cornea and reopen the aqueous leaks.
- Twenty-eight human eyes are known to have ruptured through RK incisions up to 10 years after the surgery, but no case has been documented due to diving although anecdotally one case was found at autopsy but not reported. The reported causes included accidental direct blows, assault and motor vehicle accidents.
- Corneal infection has also been reported years after the surgery was performed.
- It has been suggested that reversible increases in intraocular pressure within the mask may flatten the cornea and transiently change visual acuity so that if divers had multiple dives on consecutive days, they could experience a prolonged alteration in their visual acuity. A recent study, however, did not find any change in visual acuity or refractive error after hyperbaric exposure (Peters).
- A complication after surgery is excessive glare and halo. This might be exacerbated whilst night diving.

Consider the risk of corneal infection in the postoperative period (a plausible, remote and moderate risk).

**This risk may be reduced by waiting six weeks post-operatively before diving.**

Consider the risk of rupture of the cornea from a severe mask squeeze (a possible, rare and moderate risk).

**This risk may be reduced by delaying diving for three months after the procedure.**

**We recommend diving only after three months. We reinforce the prevention of mask squeeze and recommend that they wear goggles for normal swimming activities and keep their mask on at all times whilst diving, especially when practising "no-mask" swimming when it can just be flooded.**

**Divers should now be advised to have an excimer laser keratotomy for correction of refractive errors.**

## RETINAL DETACHMENT

- The reason for the detachment must be determined and assessed e.g., glaucoma, diabetes, aspirin, anticoagulants.
- Occasionally inert gas bubbles are used for internal compression during retinal detachment surgery. A gas such as sulphur hexafluoride (SF6) is chosen for its high molecular weight and slow dispersal rate. Diving whilst the bubble is present in the eyeball will change its volume and destabilize it.

Consider the risk of a gas bubble within the eyeball being disturbed and aggravating a retinal detachment (a possible, remote and moderate risk).

## VISUAL ACUITY

- Vision must be adequate to read gauges and locate the buddy diver and entry and exit points.
- Visual acuity can be reduced by poor light at depth.

- Commercial divers are required to have a corrected visual acuity of 6/12.

Consider the risk of poor vision compromising safety because gauges cannot be read or exit points not located.

**This risk may be reduced by the diver wearing contact lenses or a prescription mask and ensuring with their buddy that gauges are large, easily read and the dive entry and exit can be easily located. A torch can be carried for reading gauges at depth. At night special lights can be employed to help.**

**In reality, no one normally wants to dive unless they can see the underwater environment. The magnifying effect of the mask will help the effects of presbyopia. Visually impaired divers who dive for the sensation are fully aware of their disability and will have adequate support to overcome it.**

## FURTHER READING:


1. Andenmatten R, Piguet B, Klainguti G. Orbital haemorrhage induced by barotrauma (letter). Am J Ophthalmol 1994; 118: 536-537
2. Brown M S, Siegel I M. Cornea-contact lens interaction in the aquatic environment. CLAO J 1997; 23(4): 237-242
3. Butler F K. Diving and Hyperbaric Ophthalmology. 1995; 39: 347-366
4. Butler F K. High Pressure Ophthalmology. Alert Diver May/June 1998: 33-7
5. Creel D J, Crandall A S, Swartz M. Hyperopic shift induced by high altitude after radial keratotomy. J Refrect Surg 1997; 13(4): 389-400
6. Isenberg S J, Diamant A. Scuba diving after enucleation (letter). Am J Ophthal 1985; 100: 616-617
7. Josephson J E, Caffery B E. Contact lens considerations in surface and subsurface aqueous environments. Optom Vis Sci 1991; 68: 2-11
8. Kluger M. Fitness to Dive – Implications of Corneal Surgery. SPUMS J 1994; 24: 62-66
9. Le May M. Fitness To Dive – Ophthalmological Aspects. SPUMS J 1996; 26(4): 253-9
10. Meister DJ, Fisher SW. Progress in the spectacle correction of presbyopia. Part 1: Design and development of progressive lenses. Clinical and Experimental Optometry 2008; 91(3):240-50
11. Peters N T, Borer R C Jr, Strauss M B. Effect of increased atmospheric pressure on radial keratotomy. J Cataract Refract Surg 1999; 25(12): 1620-3
12. Stamler J F. The complications of contact lens wear. Curr Opin in Ophthalmology 1998; 9(4): 66-71
13. Vinger P F, Mieler W F, Oestricher J H, Easterbrook M. Ruptured Globes Following Radial and Hexagonal Keratotomy Surgery. Arch Opthalmol. 1996; 114: 129-134

# Respiratory Diseases

# 20

The lungs must be viewed from three paradigms when considering diving medicine.

## 1. Ventilatory Capacity

Any reduction in ventilation of the lungs will also reduce arterial oxygenation and exercise tolerance, whilst diving ventilatory capacity is reduced by:

- Breathing dense air
- There is a linear increase in air density with pressure. The deeper one dives, the denser the air. This causes an increased flow resistance, which reduces the maximum voluntary ventilation (MVV). At 20 m (66 feet) and 3 ATA pressure, the MVV is reduced by 35%; at 40 m (132 feet) and 5 ATA, by 50%.
- Water immersion, which changes pulmonary compliance.
- When immersed there is a redistribution of 500-800 ml of blood from the extremities into the thorax. This will engorge the pulmonary vessels, causing an increase in central venous and pulmonary artery pressures and a decrease in lung volume. Moreover, the engorged pulmonary vessels may impinge on the airways, further increasing airway resistance.

## 2. Bubble Trapping

During decompression venous bubbles are very common (Dunford). The pulmonary capillary bed acts as a "bubble trap" preventing venous bubbles from entering the arterial circulation and causing arterial gas embolism (AGE). They are then excreted through the alveoli.

Factors, other than the degree of bubbling, which may promote bubble redistribution through the pulmonary capillary bed and possibly increase the risk of decompression illness include:

- Any arterial-venous short circuit of the pulmonary circulation e.g., intrapulmonary arterial-venous (AV) anastomoses (IPAVA), intra-cardiac right to left shunts (PFO or ASD).
- Elevation of pulmonary artery pressure or decrease in mean systemic arterial pressure.
- Any drug, which causes vasodilation of the pulmonary vasculature, e.g., aminophylline, sildenafil.

## 3. Hyperinflation

- Whilst diving, should compressed gas become trapped in the lung during ascent, its expansion can cause overinflation of the lung tissue causing it to tear (pulmonary barotrauma), which may cause several life-threatening conditions, viz. arterial gas embolism (AGE), pneumothorax or mediastinal and subcutaneous emphysema. This is more likely to occur nearer the surface than at depth.

Intrapulmonary pressures as little as 60-80 mmHg have been shown to result in pulmonary barotrauma. This pressure differential can occur by a diver ascending only 1 m (3 feet) whilst holding their breath.

- Any condition, which causes air trapping or hyperinflation of the lungs, may predispose to pulmonary barotrauma.
- Any condition which causes stiffening of the lungs may predispose to pulmonary barotrauma.
- If the lung or pleura has scar tissue or is tethered by adhesions, the interface between the normal elastic lung tissue and the scar tissue will have varying lung compliance, creating regional differences in lung expansion and the normal lung tissue may be more likely to tear.

## ASTHMA

Reactive Airways Disease, Bronchospasm, Wheezing

- A 2016 review of recent literature concluded "due to limited evidence it is difficult to draw valid conclusions, but there are indications that recreational divers with asthma may be at increased risk for diving-related injuries" (Ustrup).
- However, other reviews and surveys have shown many asthmatics do dive yet they are not over-represented in the diving death statistics (Lippman, Ascensio-Lane).
- Over the past decades, it has become apparent that more than a single disease, asthma is the common label for many conditions, the common clinical expression of which is the presence of at least partially reversible airway obstruction and evidence of bronchial hyperresponsiveness (BHR) (Martinez). The challenge is to try an identify and advise those who are at increased risk.
- Asthma is sometimes associated with bronchiectasis and emphysema which does not always correlate with the severity of asthma (Silva).

The main concerns for the asthmatic diver are:

» Air trapping: asthmatics may have obstructed airways from bronchospasm, mucosal inflammation and mucus plugs reducing expiratory flow and being at extra risk for pulmonary overinflation and barotrauma.

» Bronchospasm being induced or exacerbated whilst diving: underwater the diver is exposed to many factors which may precipitate bronchial spasm; viz. exercise, cold air, dry air, anxiety with or without hyperventilation, possible inhalation of a fine mist of salt water through a faulty regulator. Even pollen has been found in a scuba tank (Asterita).

» Hyperinflated lungs: chronic asthmatics often have hyperinflated lungs causing them to breathe at higher lung volumes and therefore may be more susceptible to overinflation and pulmonary barotrauma.

» Patchy effect of bronchodilator inhalers: inhaled bronchodilator drugs may leave patchy obstruction within the bronchial tree. Bronchodilator drugs given before a dive may lose their full effect before the end of a dive.

» Effect of denser air: at depth the air breathed becomes denser and the work of breathing becomes greater. Any bronchospasm will amplify this effect.

» Earlier onset of panic: if the diver gets into any difficulty underwater, or even on the surface, and a wheeze is induced though anxiety or inspiration of seawater, it will compound the problem and panic will occur at an earlier stage than a non-asthmatic.

» Decompression illness: bronchodilator drugs could dilate the pulmonary blood vessels and predispose them to decompression illness.

Whatever the theoretical concerns, there is a significant population of asthmatics who want to dive and will not accept a blanket-like ban or a theoretical risk.

Consider the risk of air trapping predisposing to pulmonary barotrauma (a plausible, remote and major risk).

Consider the risk of acute bronchospasm being aggravated whilst diving and predisposing to pulmonary barotrauma and drowning (a plausible, remote and major risk).

Consider the risk of acute bronchospasm being aggravated whilst diving and reducing exercise tolerance whilst both underwater and, on the surface (a plausible, remote and moderate risk).

Consider the risk of decompression illness in a diver who has recently taken a bronchodilator drug (a possible, remote and moderate risk).

Consider the risk of other respiratory diseases that have not been recognized.

A thorough history and a pulmonary function test (with a bronchial provocation test if indicated) will help elucidate the status of asthma. If there is any suspicion of any other respiratory disease present, a chest X-ray or CT is recommended.

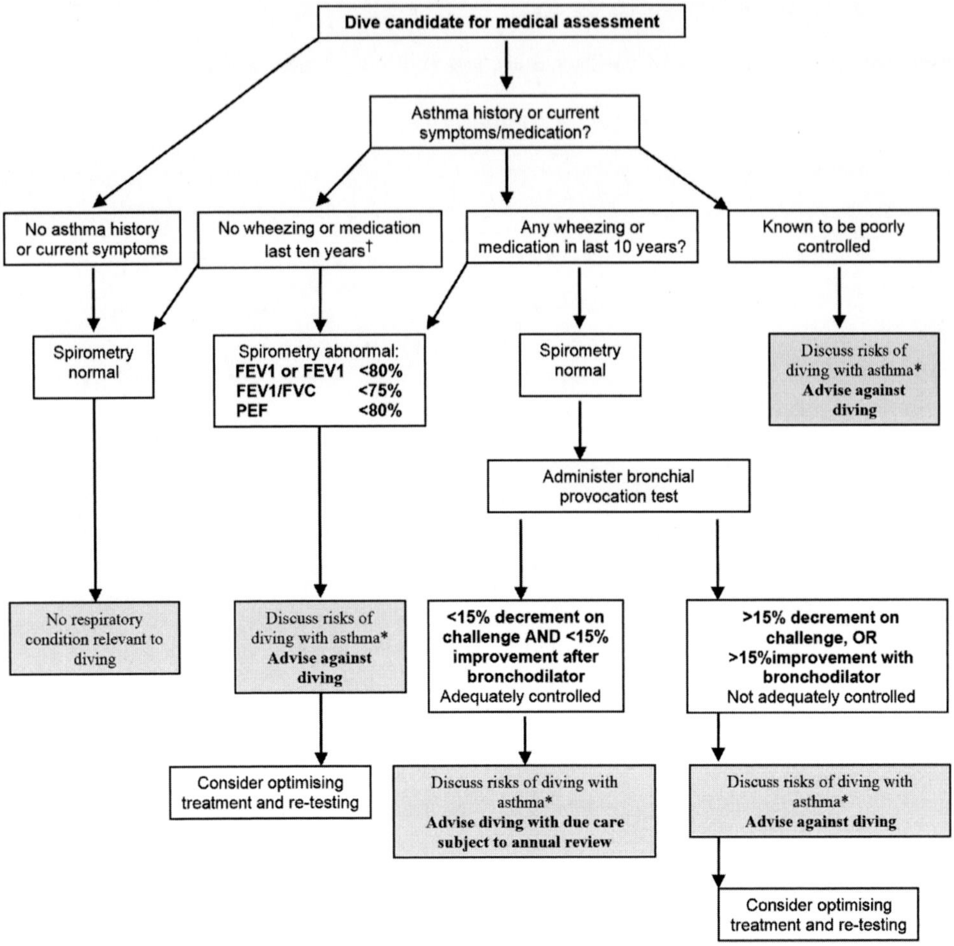


Flowchart to guide the management of fitness to dive in diving candidates with asthma. Reproduced with courtesy from the South Pacific Underwater Medicine Society 2020 guidelines on "Medical Risk Assessment for Recreational Diving".

These risks may be reduced by:

- » education of the diver to ensure they understand the potential risks and consequences of those risks whilst diving.
- » education of the diver to understand their condition and the importance of achieving excellent regular control of their asthma symptoms. If they are on preventative treatment to understand the importance of complying with their treatment.
- » regular checking of airway function using a peak flow meter for a few days before a planned dive to ensure they are 'wheeze free' (bronchospasm can be insidious, its presence is not apparent until it is relieved.)
- » emphasis on the importance of slow, controlled ascents whilst diving.
- » emphasis on the importance of ceasing diving if the level of asthma control deteriorates and any wheeze recurs.

**We recommend diving to anyone with controlled asthma on BTS step 1 or 2, only if they have a normal respiratory function and a normal bronchial provocation and/or exercise challenge test. We strongly reinforce the recommendations above to reduce the risk and especially reinforce that if their pattern of asthma changes to "persistent", they cease all diving until reassessed.**

**We do not recommend diving to anyone with cold, exercise or emotion-triggered asthma.**

**We do not recommend diving to anyone with active asthma or if they have wheezed within two months.**

We spend adequate time explaining the reasons why. If they are not on preventative treatment, we encourage them to discuss with their respiratory physician if it is appropriate for them to commence it. If this eventually controls their asthma and they become non-responsive to exercise and bronchial provocation tests, then diving may be recommended.

## IMMERSION PULMONARY OEDEMA (IPO)

- A clinical entity which has been documented since the 1980s, but which has recently come to the foreground as responsible for a subset of diving-related fatalities (Wilmshurst).
- Has a variable clinical course and severity, from transitory cough to breathlessness, haemoptysis, acute respiratory distress and even collapse, all precipitated by immersion.
- Known triggers include environmental stressors (cold temperatures, intense physical exercise, negative static lung loading) and individual susceptibilities, such as hypertension, valvular heart disease and silent coronary artery disease, obesity, female gender and advanced age.
- It has also been described in highly fit, young individuals, such as military personnel and triathlon swimmers.
- The pathophysiology involves elevated pulmonary vascular pressure, leading to interstitial alveolar oedema, brought about by central redistribution of blood volume, vasoconstriction and reduced re-absorptive capacity for excessive lung water.

Consider the risk of symptoms precipitating cardio-respiratory compromise in water.

Consider the risk of symptoms presenting at depth precipitating a rapid ascent, with its inherent risk of pulmonary barotrauma and arterial gas embolism.

Consider the risk of recurrence of immersion pulmonary oedema on re-exposure to immersion and the risk of sudden cardiac death.

**We would not advise any diver who survives one episode of documented immersion pulmonary oedema to dive again (nor breath-hold dive, nor swim).**

## COVID-19

Severe acute respiratory syndrome coronavirus 2 (SARS-CoV-2)

- An infection caused by a novel beta coronavirus, named severe acute respiratory syndrome coronavirus 2 (SARS-CoV-2), reached a pandemic status in 2020 after being discovered in Wuhan, China in late 2019, before being propagated around the globe.
- Causes an illness of variable severity, ranging from:
  - asymptomatic carriers
  - symptomatic infection with breathlessness, cough, fatigue, malaise, loss of taste and smell and altered bowel habit
  - adult respiratory distress syndrome requiring mechanical ventilation, cardiac dysfunction, pro-thrombotic tendency, neurological involvement and renal impairment.
  - Death
- Long-term follow-up is still ongoing, but it is already evident a subset of patients infected with COVID-19, despite getting over the initial infective phase, remain with longstanding symptoms, impaired exercise tolerance, fatigue, structural pulmonary parenchymal changes and respiratory function, as well as psychological sequelae, so-called "long Covid".
- Pneumonia with ground glass opacities and pulmonary embolism are well documented.

Consider the risk of lung parenchymal involvement leading to reduced exercise tolerance (a proven, remote and moderate risk).

Consider the risk of lung parenchymal involvement leading to blebs and cavitating lesions which predispose to air trapping and the inherent risk of pulmonary barotrauma (a plausible, remote and moderate risk).

Consider the risk of cardiac myocardial dysfunction predisposing to arrhythmia, impaired exercise tolerance and decreased global cardiac function (a possible, remote and major risk).

**We would only recommend asymptomatic divers to dive if they accept the risk of latent pulmonary structural changes and their remote risk of precipitating pulmonary barotrauma and arterial gas embolism. Lung imaging is at the discretion of the diving medical examiner.**

**We would not advise any diver with evidence of pulmonary, cardiac or neurological end-organ damage post-COVID-19 to dive.**

**We would screen every prospective diving candidate who had symptomatic COVID-19 with lung imaging, pulmonary function testing with dynamic spirometry and functional exercise testing, including exercise ECG, echocardiography and oximetry (do not proceed if SpO2 < 95%, a 4% decrement in SpO2 is evidence of exercise-induced desaturation).**

**Divers with symptomatic COVID-19 infection are advised to wait for a period of 3 months prior to having their fitness to dive assessed, whereas those who required hospitalisation and/or mechanical ventilation are advised to wait for a period of 6-12 months prior to having their fitness to dive assessed – respiratory and cardiology expert input is suggested and the fitness to dive assessment should be a holistic team-based assessment.**

## BRONCHIAL CARCINOMA

Lung cancer

- Lung cancer is nine per cent of all new cancers in Australia – the fifth commonest type of cancer.

- Any tumour of the lung will disrupt the architecture and obstruct the airways.
- Surgery or radiation will further disrupt the architecture and create scar tissue and pleural adhesions
- The malignant disease often causes fatigue and general malaise.
- After surgery or radiation, there will be a significant reduction in exercise tolerance.

Consider the risk of increased pulmonary barotrauma due to abnormal lung architecture, scar tissue and adhesions (a possible, remote and major risk).

Consider the risk of reduction in exercise tolerance (a proven, regular and moderate risk).

**We would not recommend diving to anyone with this history.**

## CHEST SURGERY

Thoracotomy, Intrathoracic surgery

- The reason for the surgery needs to be determined and assessed.
- After any surgery where the pleura has been opened, there will be possible adhesions between the chest wall and the visceral pleura.
- Any surgery to the lung itself will leave scar tissue, which is less compliant than a normal lung.

Consider the risk from the underlying condition requiring surgery.

Consider the risk of pleural adhesions and pulmonary scar tissue predisposing to pulmonary barotrauma (a possible, remote and major risk).

**This risk may be reduced by explaining the possible dangers to the diver and emphasizing the importance of a slow ascent rate whilst diving.**

A high-resolution spiral lung CT scan may show the extent of scarring, adhesions and presence of any air trapping, but does not equate to a certainty about fitness to dive.

**If the surgery did not open the lung itself but just went into the pleural cavity, we do not discourage diving but will reinforce the importance of a slow ascent rate.**

**If the surgery involved the lung parenchyma, we would strongly discourage diving.**

## CHEST WALL INJURIES

Crushed chest, Multiple rib fractures

- Often this type of injury is associated with a traumatic penetrating pneumothorax and haemothorax, with a high probability of scarring to the pleura and peripheral lung tissue, with adhesions between the visceral pleura and chest wall.
- Treatment may have involved intrapleural chest drains and mechanical ventilation. The extent of the damage and any complications e.g., adult respiratory distress syndrome, need to be determined and assessed.

Consider the risk of pleural adhesions and pulmonary scar tissue predisposing to pulmonary barotrauma (a possible, remote and major risk).

**This risk may be reduced by explaining the possible dangers to the diver and emphasizing the importance of a**

**slow ascent rate whilst diving. A high-resolution spiral lung CT scan may show the extent of scarring, adhesions and presence of any air trapping.**

Consider the risk of any medical complications e.g., adult respiratory distress syndrome.

**If there is the involvement of lung parenchyma, we would strongly discourage diving.**

## CHRONIC OBSTRUCTIVE PULMONARY DISEASE (COPD)

Emphysema, Chronic Bronchitis

- Emphysema is characterized by abnormal enlargement of the air spaces distal to the terminal bronchioles, with the destruction of alveolar walls and the formation of bullae.
- It causes obstruction by decreasing the lung's elastic recoil, which normally holds the airways open in expiration.
- Chronic bronchitis is characterized by increased mucus-producing cells in the walls of the bronchi and bronchioles and causes obstruction by narrowing the small airway passages with mucosal thickening and mucus plugs.
- Lung function tests will show an obstructive pattern with a low FEV1/FVC ratio and the chest X-ray shows hyperinflation.
- Some people with COPD will retain carbon dioxide. Although such patients are unlikely to present themselves for diving this may predispose them to carbon dioxide toxicity and oxygen toxicity and enhance nitrogen narcosis.
- Many people with COPD will be taking regular bronchodilators.

Consider the risk of reduced exercise tolerance (a proven, regular and moderate risk).

Consider the risk of increased pulmonary barotrauma (a plausible, regular and major risk).

Consider the risk of carbon dioxide toxicity and nitrogen narcosis (a possible, regular and moderate risk).

Consider the risk of increased incidence of decompression illness from the recent use of bronchodilators (a possible, remote and moderate risk).

**We would not recommend anyone with COPD to dive. We consider it a total contraindication to compressed gas diving.**

## EXTRINSIC ALLERGIC ALVEOLITIS

e.g., Farmer's lung, Bird Fancier's Lung, Mushroom Worker Lung, Pituitary Snuff Taker's Lung, Thatched Roof Lung, Woodworker's Lung

- This is a chronic inflammatory disease of the lung, resulting from sensitization and subsequent exposure to a variety of foreign proteins, e.g., spores from microorganisms or low-weight molecular chemicals.
- An acute attack occurs 4-8 hours after exposure causing fever, malaise, dry cough and dyspnoea.
- Chronic disease may follow as few as five acute recurrences leading to significantly reduced lung function.
- The chronic form may become progressive and result in progressive respiratory failure.

Consider the risk of reduced exercise tolerance (a plausible, regular and moderate risk).

**This risk can be reduced by waiting until lung function and exercise tolerance have returned to normal after an acute attack.**

Consider the risk of increased pulmonary barotrauma (a possible, remote and major risk).

**This risk may be reduced by a chest X-ray to ensure that the chronic features of pulmonary fibrosis are absent.**

**We recommend that divers wait at least four weeks after an acute attack. Anyone with a history of recurrent attacks we refer for a full respiratory assessment, including imaging and spirometry.**

## PLEURAL ADHESIONS

- They will tether the visceral pleura to the chest wall or the diaphragm reducing the elasticity of the underlying lung tissue.
- The tethered lung tissue may tear at a lesser degree of hyperinflation than normal lung tissue.
- Experimentally diaphragmatic pleural adhesions were demonstrated to cause more pulmonary barotrauma than pleural adhesions to the chest wall (Malhotra).
- One study reporting autopsy on divers after fatal pulmonary barotrauma noted that lung damage was not always located around scars and foci of pulmonary fibrosis, but may occur distant to the scar as the scar changed the architecture such that the tear occurred at a weaker site (Calder).

Consider the risks of increased incidence of pulmonary barotrauma (a plausible, remote and major risk).

**This risk may be reduced by explaining the possible dangers to the diver and emphasizing the importance of a slow ascent rate whilst diving. A high-resolution spiral lung CT scan may show the extent of scarring, adhesions and presence of any air trapping (Knisely).**

**If there are extensive adhesions, we strongly discourage diving.**

## PNEUMOTHORAX - SPONTANEOUS

- It normally reflects an underlying cystic lung disease, usually the rupture of a subpleural bleb or bulla. Most occur during periods of light physical activity or sleep.
- They typically occur in thin tall males aged 20-29 but this is not exclusive.
- There is a recurrence rate of 30-50% when just breathing air at atmospheric pressures. There is no data on recurrence rate due to diving because it has always been considered a contraindication to diving.
- A secondary spontaneous pneumothorax is caused by many lung diseases including asthma, scleroderma, tuberous sclerosis and chronic obstructive airway disease.
- A pneumothorax occurring underwater will increase in size on ascent causing tension and cardiac impairment, with potentially catastrophic consequences.

Consider the risk of a recurrent pneumothorax occurring due to hyperinflation of a small subpleural bulla (a plausible, regular and major risk).

**This risk may be reduced by excluding obvious pulmonary cystic disease with a high-definition spiral lung CT scan (but will not exclude all cysts).**

**We would not recommend anyone with this condition to dive. We consider it a total contraindication to compressed gas diving.**

## PNEUMOTHORAX - TRAUMATIC

- Usually caused by a penetrating chest injury, which will leave some scarring and pleural adhesions.
- It may be caused by blunt injury to the chest wall or by mechanical ventilation of the lungs.

Consider the risk of pleural adhesions and pulmonary scar tissue predisposing to pulmonary barotrauma (a possible, remote and major risk).

**This risk may be reduced by explaining the possible dangers to the diver and emphasizing the importance of a slow ascent rate whilst diving. A high-resolution spiral lung CT scan may show the extent of scarring, adhesions and presence of any air trapping.**

## PLEURODESIS & PLEURECTOMY

- Commonly performed for recurrent primary spontaneous pneumothorax (PSP).
- Recurrence rates of up to 8% following the procedures have been cited, but it is difficult to assess recurrence rate seeing the different procedures used, e.g., talc pleurodesis, abrasion of the parietal pleura only or bilateral surgical pleurectomy via thoracoscopy or VATS (Germonpre).
- Recurrence after a pleurectomy has been documented, due to the formation of neo-pleura by mesenchymal cells not removed entirely during the procedure (Germonpre).
- There is a high probability of therapeutically-induced pulmonary scarring as well as an underlying cystic lung disease. These may cause pulmonary barotrauma, possibly causing an arterial gas embolism (AGE).

Consider the risk of pulmonary barotrauma (a possible, rare and major risk).

**We would very strongly discourage anyone to dive after both of these procedures.**

## PNEUMOCONIOSES

Silicosis, Coal Worker's pneumoconiosis, Talcosis, Volcanic Ash Lung

- This is caused by mineral dust irritation of the lungs leading to pulmonary fibrosis. Progressive, massive fibrosis may occur with cavitation.
- In the early stages, there may be no symptoms despite chest X-ray changes.
- Asbestos exposure can cause benign pleural effusions, calcified pleural plaques, asbestosis and mesothelioma.

Consider the risk of pulmonary barotrauma due to the reduced compliance of the lungs (a plausible, regular to remote, major risk).

**This risk may be reduced by first fully assessing the lung with a high-definition spiral lung CT scan.**

Consider the risk of reduced exercise tolerance (a proven, regular and moderate risk).

**This risk may be reduced by an assessment of exercise tolerance to ensure an adequate level of physical fitness. If reduced, a supervised exercise program may increase exercise tolerance to an acceptable level.**

**We would not normally recommend anyone with this condition to dive.**

## PULMONARY ARTERIOVENOUS FISTULA (PAVF)

e.g., Rendu Osler Weber disease, Anomalous pulmonary venous drainage

- The pulmonary venous/capillary bed acts as a filter for bubbles in the venous circulation. Any arterio-venous fistula will act as a bypass and allow bubbles to enter the arterial vasculature.

Consider the risk of increased incidence of decompression illness (a possible, remote and moderate risk).

**We would not recommend anyone with this condition to dive.**

## PULMONARY CYSTS & BULLAE

- Any cavity in the lung which traps air will be at risk of causing pulmonary barotrauma. Many cysts are congenital and the diver is completely unaware of their existence.
- Cysts may not be apparent on chest X-ray, only seen on high-resolution CT of the thorax (Goffinet).
- The cyst may rupture and cause pneumothorax or become tensioned and enlarge causing chest pain (Simpson).
- Fatalities have been reported from arterial gas embolism (AGE) (Zaug).

Consider the risk of air trapping and pulmonary barotrauma (a plausible, remote and major risk).

**We would not recommend diving to anyone with a lung cyst or bulla. We would consider it a contraindication to diving.**

## PULMONARY EMBOLUS (PE)

- If no infarction has occurred, the architecture and structure of the lung are preserved and resolution should result in normal lung tissue.
- If infarction occurs there may be some scarring and adhesions. Occasionally it can lead to pulmonary hypertension and reduced cardiac output restricting exercise tolerance.
- The cause of PE needs to be established. If it was derived from a DVT, what was its cause? If it was idiopathic is there a danger of recurrent embolism? Some patients with recurrent DVT and PE are anticoagulated.

Consider the risk of pulmonary hypertension restricting exercise tolerance (a plausible, rare and moderate risk).

**This risk may be reduced by prior cardiological assessment.**

Consider the risk of increased incidence of pulmonary barotrauma from scarring and adhesions (a possible, rare and major risk).

**This risk may be reduced by a high-definition spiral CT lung scan excluding air trapping.**

**If there are no complications six months following the PE, exercise tolerance is normal and the high-definition spiral CT lung scan is also normal, then we recommend diving.**

## SARCOIDOSIS

- This multisystem granulomatous disease commonly affects the lung.
- Pulmonary sarcoidosis can be symptomless and only found on routine chest X-rays which may show mediastinal lymphadenopathy and parenchymal infiltrates.
- Abnormalities on chest X-rays are present in 90-95% of all cases.
- Spontaneous remission occurs in two-thirds of all cases. Ninety per cent of patients with radiographic stage one disease spontaneously remit.
- Eighty-five per cent of remissions occur within the first two years.
- A case of decompression illness in a hyperbaric chamber has been attributed to asymptomatic sarcoidosis (Tetzlaff).

Consider the risk of pulmonary infiltrates increasing the incidence of pulmonary barotrauma (a plausible, remote and major risk).

The risk can be reduced by a full respiratory assessment prior to diving to ensure full remission. Even after remission, another assessment after one year is advised.

**Once remission has occurred, we recommend diving.**

### Adult respiratory distress syndrome (ARDS)

- An acute, progressive respiratory failure that usually follows severe trauma.
- Even after apparent recovery, reduced lung compliance can continue.
- Subpleural air cysts and pulmonary fibrosis are common long-term sequelae.

Consider the risk of increased incidence of pulmonary barotrauma because of pulmonary fibrosis or subpleural cysts (a proven, rare and major risk).

Consider the risk of reduced exercise tolerance because of pulmonary fibrosis (a probable, remote and moderate risk).

**We would not recommend anyone with this history until they had had a normal high-resolution spiral lung CT scan and a full assessment by a respiratory physician.**

## SLEEP APNOEA, OBSTRUCTIVE

- This causes apnoeic/hyponeic/hypoxic periods whilst asleep, resulting in disturbed and unrefreshing sleep. It results in daytime sleepiness, fatigue, irritability and poor concentration.
- It is often associated with obesity and poor physical fitness.
- It is a risk factor for hypertension. It can lead to depression, cardiomyopathy and pulmonary hypertension (Roux).
- The long frequent apnoeic periods whilst sleeping may cause carbon dioxide retention and physiological acclimatization to high carbon dioxide levels may occur. This may predispose the diver to the risks of carbon dioxide toxicity, unusual degrees of nitrogen narcosis or susceptibility to oxygen toxicity.
- Continuous positive airway pressure (CPAP) via a nasal mask during sleep is the best treatment but does not help all cases.

Consider the risk of decreased concentration and fatigue predisposing to lack of care and attention leading to accidents (a plausible, regular and moderate risk).

Consider the risk of carbon dioxide toxicity, nitrogen narcosis and oxygen toxicity (a possible, remote and moderate risk).

**This risk may be reduced by limiting the depth of diving to only diving in very sheltered and calm conditions where it is less likely to have heavy exercise such as hard finning.**

Consider the risk of associated hypertension and heart disease.

Consider the risks of obesity and poor physical fitness.

**If the diver has no cardiovascular complications, has a normal exercise tolerance, is being treated with CPAP and is symptom-free, we would recommend diving. If there has been a significant history of moderate to severe sleep apnoea, we suggest a depth limitation of 18 m (60 ft).**

## TRACHEOSTOMY – NOW CLOSED

- The reason for which the tracheostomy was performed needs to be reviewed.
- The method of tracheostomy should be assessed. The Bjork method can lead to the inspiratory collapse of the trachea,

especially when hyperventilating and limiting exercise tolerance. A midline slit of the trachea heals more rigidly.

- The upper airway is not the limiting factor for expiratory flow rates. A slightly narrowed trachea will not be a risk factor for pulmonary barotrauma.

Consider the risks, if any, of the reason for the tracheostomy to be performed.

Consider the risk of inspiratory collapse of the tracheostomy scar-limiting exercise tolerance.

**To check for inspiratory collapse, ask the diver to hyperventilate for 20 breaths and listen for any stridor.**

## FURTHER READING:


1. Adir Y, Bove AA. Can asthmatic subjects dive? Eur Respir Rev 2016 Jun;25(140):214-20. doi: 10.1183/16000617.0006-2016. PMID: 27246598

2. Anderson S D, Brannan J B, Trevillion L, Young H. Lung function and Bronchial Provocation Tests for Intending Divers with a history of asthma. SPUMS J 1995; 25940: 233-48

3. Ascencio-Lane JC, Smart D, Lippmann J. A twenty-year analysis of compressed gas diving-related deaths in Tasmania. Diving and Hyperbaric Medicine. 2019 March 31;49(1):21–29. doi: 10.28920/dhm49.1.21-29. PMID: 30856664.

4. Ashrafi R, Turner M. Pulmonary barotrauma: assessment and investigation in divers. Undersea Hyperb Med 2019 Mar-Apr-May;46:189-196. PMID: 31051064

5. Astarita C, Gargano D, Di-Martino P. Pollen trapped in a scuba tank: a potential hazard for allergic divers (letter). Ann Intern Med 2000; 132(2): 166-7

6. Bar Or O, Inbar O. Swimming and asthma. Benefits and deleterious effects. Sports Med 1992; 14(6): 397-40

7. Bonnemaison B, Castagna O, de Maistre S, Blatteau JE. Chest CT scan for the screening of air anomalies at risk of pulmonary barotrauma for the initial medical assessment of fitness to dive in a military population. Front Physiol. 2022 Oct 7;13:1005698. doi: 10.3389/fphys.2022.1005698. eCollection 2022. PMID: 36277200, PMCID: PMC9585318

8. Boussuges A, Chaumet G. Hypertension and risk of immersion pulmonary oedema. Int J Cardiol 2014 Jul 1;174(3):873. doi: 10.1016/j.ijcard.2014.04.210. Epub 2014 Apr 28. PMID: 24820747

9. Bove A. Observations on asthma in the recreational diving population. SPUMS J 1995; 25(4): 225

10. Brooks G, Pethybridge R J, Pearson R R. Lung function reference values from FEV1, FVC, FEV1/FVC ratio and FEF(25-75) derived from the results of screening 3788 Royal Navy submariners and submariner candidates by spirometry. Proceedings of the XIVth Annual Meeting of the European Undersea Biomedical Society, Aberdeen, Scotland 1988. Reprinted in SPUMS J 1990; 20(3): 187-94

11. Boussuges A, Ayme K, Chaumet G, Albier E, Borgnetta M, Gavarry O. Observational study of potential risk factors of immersion pulmonary oedema in healthy divers: exercise intensity is the main contributor. Sports Med Open 2017 Oct 3;3(1):35. doi: 10.1186/s40798-017-0104-1. PMID: 28975560 PMCID: PMC5626674

12. Calder I M. Autopsy and experimental observations on factors leading to barotrauma in man. Undersea Biomed Res 1985; 12(2): 165-82

13. Castagna O, Gempp E, Poyet R, Schmid B, Desruelle AV, Crunel V, Maurin A, Choppard R, MacIver DH. Cardiovascular Mechanisms of Extravascular Lung Water Accumulation in Divers. Am J Cardiol 2017 Mar 15;119(6):929-932. doi: 10.1016/j.amjcard.2016.11.050. Epub 2017 Jan 20. PMID: 28189252

14. Castagna O, Regnard J, Gempp E, Louge P, Brocq FX, Schmid B, Desruelle AV, Crunel V, Maurin A, Chopard R, MacIver

DH. The Key Roles of Negative Pressure Breathing and Exercise in the Development of Interstitial Pulmonary Oedema in Professional Male SCUBA Divers. Sports Med Open 2018 Jan 3;4(1):1. doi: 10.1186/s40798-017-0116-x. PMID: 29299780 PMCID: PMC5752643

15. Colebatch H J H, Smith M M, Ng C K Y. Increased elastic recoil as a determinant of pulmonary barotrauma in divers. Respir Physiol 1976; 26: 55-64

16. Coop CA, Adams KE, Webb CN. SCUBA Diving and Asthma: Clinical Recommendations and Safety. Clin Rev Allergy Immunol 2016 Feb;50(1):18-22. doi: 10.1007/s12016-015-8474-y.

17. Coulange M, Rossi P, Gargne O, Gole Y, Bessereau J, Regnard J, Jammes Y, Barthelemy A, Auffray JP, Boussuges A. Pulmonary oedema in healthy SCUBA divers: new physiopathological pathways. Clin Physiol Funct Imaging 2010 May;30(3):181-6. doi: 10.1111/j.1475-097X.2010.00922.x. Epub 2010 Feb 4. PMID: 20141520 DOI: 10.1111/j.1475-097X.2010.00922.x

18. Curson K S, Dovenbarger J A, Moon R E, Hodder S, Bennett P B. Risk assessment of asthma for decompression illness. Undersea Biomed Res 1991; 18(Suppl): 16

19. Davies MJ, Fisher LH, Chegini S, Craig TJ. Asthma and the diver. Clin Rev Allergy Immunol 2005 Oct;29(2):131-8. doi: 10.1385/CRIAI:29:2:131.

20. De Bakker HM, Tijsterman M, de Bakker-Teunissen OJG, Soerdjbalie-Maikoe V, van Hulst RA, de Bakker BS. Prevalence of Pulmonary Bullae and Blebs in Postmortem CT Imaging with Potential Implications for Diving Medicine. Chest 2020 Apr;157(4):916-923. doi: 10.1016/j.chest.2019.11.008. Epub 2019 Nov 22. PMID: 31759963

21. Edmonds C, Walker D. Scuba diving fatalities in Australia and New Zealand; 1. The human factor. SPUMS J 1989; 19(3): 94-104

22. Elliot D H (ed). Are Asthmatics Fit To Dive? Symposia at UHMS Annual Meeting, June 1995. Undersea and Hyperbaric Medical Society, 10531 Metropolitan Avenue, Kensington, MD 20895-2627

23. Etzlaff K, Reuter M, Kampen J, Lott C. Hyperbaric chamber-related decompression illness in a patient with asymptomatic pulmonary sarcoidosis. Aviat Space Environ Med 1999; 70(6): 594-7

24. Farrell P J S, Glanvill P. Diving practices of scuba divers with asthma. Brit Med J 1990; 300: 166

25. Francis J. Pulmonary barotrauma: a new look at mechanisms. SPUMS J 1997; 27(4): 205-18

26. Gempp E, Demaistre S, Louge P. Hypertension is predictive of recurrent immersion pulmonary oedema in scuba divers. Int J Cardiol 2014 Mar 15;172(2):528-9. doi: 10.1016/j.ijcard.2014.01.021. Epub 2014 Jan 22. PMID: 24485632

27. Germonpre P, Van Renterghem E, Dechamps N, Onghena T, Van Aken J. Recurrence of spontaneous pneumothorax six years after VATS pleurectomy: evidence for the formation of neo pleura. J Cardiothorac Surg 2020 Jul 28;15(1):191. doi: 10.1186/s13019-020-01233-9. PMID: 32723348 PMCID: PMC7389453

28. Goffinet CMJ, Simpson G. Cerebral arterial gas embolism in a scuba diver with a primary lung bulla. Diving and Hyperbaric Medicine. 2019 June 30;49(2):141–144. doi: 10.28920/dhm49.2.141-144. PMID: 31177521

29. Gore MD, Dixon G, Stantan AE. Is it safe to SCUBA dive with asthma? Expert Rev Respir Med 2019 Nov;13(11):1069-1077. doi: 10.1080/17476348.2019.1666003. Epub 2019 Sep 11. PMID: 31509025

30. Gorman D. Asthma and diving. A review of emergent attitudes and society policies. The Undersea Journal, First Quarter, 1996, 81-86

31. Gorman D, Veale A. SPUMS Policy on Asthma and Fitness for Diving. SPUMS J 1995; 25(4): 213-4

32. Hampson N B, Dunford R G. Pulmonary oedema of scuba divers. Undersea Hyperb Med 1997; 24(1): 29-33

33. Henckes A, Cochard G, Gatineau F, Louge P, Gempp E, Demaistre S, Nowak E, Ozier Y. Risk factors for immersion pulmonary edema in recreational scuba divers: a case-control study. Undersea Hyperb Med 2019;46(5):611-618. PMID: 31683358

34. Jenkins C, Anderson S D, Wong R, Veale A. Compressed air diving and respiratory disease. A discussion document of the Thoracic Society of Australia and New Zealand. Med J Aust 1993; 158: 275-9

35. Knisely B L, Kuhlnan J E. Radiographic and computer (CT) imaging of complex pleural disease. Crit Rev Diagn Imaging 1997; 38(1): 1-58 Moon R, Bryant S. Diving and the lung. SPUM J 1997; 27(4): 218-28

36. Kumar M, Thompson PD. A literature review of immersion pulmonary oedema. Phys Sportsmed 2019

37. Lippmann J, Taylor D McD. Medical conditions in scuba diving fatality victims in Australia, 2001 to 2013. Diving and Hyperbaric Medicine. 2020 June 30;50(2):98–104. doi: 10.28920/dhm50.2.98-104. PMID: 32557410.

38. Malhotra M S, Wright H C. The effects of raised intrapulmonary pressure on the lungs of fresh unchilled cadavers. J Path Bact 1962; 82: 198-202

39. Martinez FD. Beyond the Paradigm of Asthma as an Inflammatory Disease. A Summary of the 2015 Aspen Lung Conference. Annals of the American Thoracic Society, Volume 13, Issue Supplement 1

40. Mirasoglu B, Yetis G, Erelel M, Toklu AS. Post COVID-19 fitness to dive assessment findings in occupational and recreational divers. Diving Hyperb Med. 2022 Mar 31;52(1):35-43. doi: 10.28920/dhm52.1.35-43. PMID: 35313371, PMCID: PMC9177431 (available on 2023-03-31)

41. Moon RE. Immersion pulmonary oedema: drowning from the inside. Undersea Hyperb Med 2019 Sep-Dec - Fourth Quarter;46(5):577-579. PMID: 31683355

42. Ng A, Edmonds C. Immersion pulmonary oedema and Takotsubo cardiomyopathy. Diving Hyperb Med 2015 Dec;45(4):255-7. PMID: 26687314

43. Neuman T S, Bove A A, O'Connor, Kelsen S G. Asthma and diving. Annals Allergy, 1994; 73 : 344-50

44. Packham S, Ebden P. Recent advances in the sleep apnoea/hypopnoea syndrome. Hosp med 2000; 61(2): 108-11

45. Parker J. Asthma and Diving (letter). SPUMS J 1992; 22(3): 160-1

46. Prefaut C. Dubois F, Amaral-Marques R, Macklem P, Ruff F. Influence of immersion to the neck in water on airway closure and distribution of perfusion in man. Respir Physiol 1979; 37: 312-23

47. Roux F. D'Ambrosio C, Mohsenin V. Sleep-related breathing disorders and cardiovascular disease. Am J Med 2000; 108(5): 396-402

48. Ronnestad I, Thorsen E, Segadal K, Hope A. Bronchial response to breathing dry gas as 3.7 Mpa ambient pressure. Eur J Appl Physiol 1994; 69(1): 32-5

49. Sadler C, Villela MA, Van Hoesen K, Grover I, Lang M, Neuman T, Lindholm P. Diving after SARS-CoV-2 (COVID-19) infection: Fitness to dive assessment and medical guidance. Diving Hyperb Med 2020 Sep 30;50(3):278-287. doi: 10.28920/dhm50.3.278-287. PMID: 32957131 PMCID: PMC7755459

50. San Diego guidance on assessing fitness to diving for divers post COVID-19. https://health.ucsd.edu/coronavirus/Documents/UC%20San%20Diego%20Guidelines%20for%20Evaluation%20of%20Divers%20during%20COVID-19%20pandemic.pdf

51. Simpson G. Primary Lung Bullae and Scuba Diving. SPUMS J 1998; 28(1): 10-2

52. Smart D, Sage M, Davis FM. Two fatal cases of immersion pulmonary oedema - using dive accident investigation to assist the forensic pathologist. Diving Hyperb Med 2014 Jun;44(2):97-100. PMID: 24986728

53. Turner M, Benton P J. Three cases of pneumomediastinum – after labour, sneezing and compressed air diving. J R SOC Med 1998; 91(5): 268-9

54. Silva CIS, Thomas V. Colby TV, Müller NL. Asthma and Associated Conditions: High-Resolution CT and Pathologic Findings American Journal of Roentgenology, September 2004, Volume 183, Number 3

55. Swanson K L, Prakasl V B, Stanson A W. Pulmonary arteriovenous fistulas: Mayo Clinic Experience 1987-97. Maya Clinic Proc 1999; 74(7): 771-80

56. Taylor DR, Cowan JO, Greene JM, Willan AR, Sears MR. Asthma in remission: can relapse in early adulthood be predicted at 18 years of age? Chest. 2005 Mar;127(3):845-50. doi: 10.1378/chest.127.3.845.

57. Tetzlaff K, Muth CM, Waldhauser LK. A review of asthma and scuba diving. J Asthma 2002 Oct;39(7):557-66. doi: 10.1081/jas-120014920.

58. UKSDMC guidance on assessing fitness to diving for divers post COVID-19. http://www.ukdmc.org/medical-conditions/coronavirus-covid-19/

59. Ustrup AS, Ulrik CS. Are recreational SCUBA divers with asthma at increased risk? J Asthma. 2017 Oct;54(8):784-791. doi: 10.1080/02770903.2016.1263861. PMID: 27905823

60. Veale A. A Respiratory Physicians Approach to Asthma and Diving. SPUMS J 1995; 25(4): 225-30

61. Villela MA, Dunworth S, Harlan NP, Moon RE. Can my patient dive after a first episode of primary spontaneous pneumothorax? A systematic review of the literature. Undersea Hyperb Med Mar-Apr 2018;45(2):199-208. PMID: 29734572

62. Weiss LD, Van Meter KW. Cerebral air embolism in asthmatic divers in a swimming pool. Chest 1995; 107: 1653-54

63. Wilmshurst P T, Nuri M, Crowther A, Webb-Peploe M M. Cold-induced pulmonary oedema in scuba divers and swimmers and subsequent development of hypertension. Lancet 1989; 1: 62-65

64. Wilmshurst PT. Immersion pulmonary oedema: a cardiological perspective. Diving Hyperb Med 2019 Mar 31;49(1):30-40. doi: 10.28920/dhm49.1.30-40. PMID: 30856665 PMCID: PMC6526048

65. Zaugg M, Kaplan V, Widmer U, Baumann P C, Russi E W. Fatal air embolism in an airplane passenger with a giant intrapulmonary bronchogenic cyst. Am J Respir Crit Care Med 1998; 157 (5): 1686-9

# Surgical Issues

# 21

## HERNIA OF THE ABDOMINAL WALL

e.g., inguinal hernia, incisional hernia, umbilical hernia

- Diving involves lifting heavy equipment such as cylinders, weight belts and rebreathers, which could aggravate an existing hernia.
- If the hernia contains any intestine into which intestinal gas could enter during the dive, there is a possibility that on ascent the gas would expand and cause impaction, strangulation or even rupture under the influence of Boyle's law.

Consider the risks of impaction/strangulation/rupture if the hernia contains an air-filled intestine.

Consider the risk of aggravating the hernia by lifting.

**This risk may be reduced by emphasizing correct lifting techniques and avoiding heavy lifting when possible.**

**We discourage diving to anyone with a hernia until it has been surgically repaired and the subsequent healing and rehabilitation are complete.**

## KIDNEY TRANSPLANT

- It takes about a year to fully assess the result of a renal transplant. Renal function may be compromised and remain compromised.
- Patients who suffer chronic renal failure are prone to develop ischaemic heart disease prematurely and which progresses more rapidly.
- The diver is immunocompromised, usually stabilized on a maintenance regime using a triple combination of a calcineurin inhibitor (CNI) e.g., tacrolimus (Tac), an antimetabolite e.g. mycophenolate mofetil (MMK) and a corticosteroid e.g. prednisolone. Patients with a low immunological risk may only be on dual therapy where the corticosteroid is ceased.
- The common immunosuppressant drugs have no specific adverse drug reactions (ADR) relevant to diving but commonly cause nausea, diarrhoea, general malaise, headache, dizziness, tremor and paraesthesia. Toxic effects may result in neutropenia and thrombocytopenia presenting as unexplained viral, fungal and bacterial infections, mouth ulcers, bruising and bleeding.
- Prednisone can predispose to oxygen toxicity but this is only relevant to sports diving should the diver need recompression treatment, if pure oxygen is used for accelerated decompression purposes or if deep diving is entertained.
- Diabetes is a common post-transplant complication.
- The transplanted kidney is situated in the lower abdomen and could be more prone to injury from a direct blow to the abdomen.

- Patients who suffer chronic renal failure are prone to develop ischaemic heart disease prematurely and which progresses more rapidly.
- Blood pressure may be elevated or controlled with hypertension drugs.

Consider the risks of elevated blood pressure and the presence of ischaemic heart disease or diabetes.

Consider the risk of adverse drug reactions from the immunosuppressive drugs.

Consider the risk of respiratory infections being caused by contaminated water, regulator or buoyancy compensator.

**We recommend waiting for one year post-transplant before assessment. If there are no significant adverse or toxic drug effects, and renal function and blood pressure are normal, we recommend diving with caution and having an annual diving medical assessment.**

## PLASTIC SURGERY IMPLANTS

- Implants containing air spaces e.g., porous polyethylene, are used in the chin, cheek, nose and skin. As the implant wound heals the air is absorbed and invaded by fibro-neovascular tissue. By the time of full healing, all air should be replaced and there would be little danger of barotrauma, provided all air has been resorbed.

## RECENT ABDOMINAL SURGERY

- The underlying reason for the surgery needs to be reviewed.
- Major abdominal surgery can be debilitating requiring a prolonged period of convalescence to regain stamina and conditioning.
- Abdominal wounds need to be fully healed before heavy lifting is recommended. Abdominal scars need to be fully healed to avoid infection.

Consider the risks of the condition for which surgery was performed.

Consider the risk of poor exercise tolerance and easy fatigue following major surgery.

**This risk may be reduced by completing a supervised exercise program prior to resuming diving.**

Consider the risk of aggravating an incisional hernia by heavy lifting.

Consider the risk of wound infection

**We recommend a 6–8 weeks delay before diving is recommenced. If there were surgical complications e.g., wound infection or anaemia, this period should be extended. Diving should not be the first form of physical exercise performed after surgery.**

## TESTICULAR IMPLANTS

- One study tested the implant to 90m depth when singular bubbles were noted on decompression. All dives to 50 m were clear.

## FURTHER READING:


1. Kalluri HV, Karen L Hardinger KL. Current state of renal transplant immunosuppression: Present and future. World J Transplant. 2012 Aug 24; 2(4): 51–68. doi: 10.5500/wjt.v2.i4.5, PMCID: PMC3782235
2. Peusch-Dreyer D, Ahrens J, Dreyer K-H, Bosbach H, Mannche K H. Testicle implants – Diving exposure. (Abst) Underwater Hyper Med 1997; 13(3): 285

# Women & Diving

# 22

## CONTRACEPTION

The oral contraceptive pill (OCP)

- Many women use the OCP to regulate the frequency of their menstrual cycle and avoid menstruation/withdrawal bleeds when diving.
- There is no evidence that OCPs make women more susceptible to decompression illness.

## GYNAECOLOGICAL SURGERY

- Where the cervical canal has been forcibly dilated and the lining of the uterus disrupted there could be an increased risk of infection.

Consider the risk of endometritis and pelvic infection (a plausible, remote and moderate risk).

**This risk may be reduced by delaying diving until the uterine tissue hashealed. A two-week delay is recommended before diving.**

## HORMONE REPLACEMENT (HRT)

- Oestrogen patches may be more firmly applied to the skin for the duration of the dive but there is no evidence to suggest significant sudden increases in serum levels.
- Subcutaneous hormone implants will not be affectedwhilst diving.

## MAMMARY IMPLANTS / BREAST IMPLANTS

- Studies have shown that bubbles can form in both saline and silicone implants but are tolerated quite safely and without symptoms during normal recreational diving.
- Buoyancy compensators with constrictive chest straps should be avoided to prevent undue stress on the implant.
- Silicone implants are negatively buoyant and if large could alter the diver's trim in the water.

## MENSTRUAL PERIOD

- Symptoms during menstruation may include severe abdominal cramping andbloating, nausea, vomiting, headaches and fatigue. The abdominal cramping can be disabling. However, many women have reported that diving whilst experiencing period pains noticeably reduced their pain.

- Premenstrual tension may cause irritability, lethargy, emotional lability, breast tenderness and decreased mental alertness which may interfere with clear thinking.
- In one recent study, women reported an increased incidence of problems during their dives for the week before and the week following their menstrual period (St Leger Dowse).
- Severe fluid retention during the menstrual cycle could theoretically predispose to decompression illness and difficulty in equalization of the middle ear. Paradoxically a Doppler study for patency of pre-existing PFOs during the menstrual cycle showed them to manifest mid-cycle (Klein).
- The average amount of blood lost during an hour's dive whilst menstruating would only be a few millilitres, insufficient to contaminate the seawater, especially if a tampon and wetsuit are worn. Any suggestion that there is an increased risk of shark attack is completely unfounded.
- Diving during menstruation is quite possible but requires some adjustments, especially for everything related to changes of protection during the day (not always obvious on a boat or during two tank dives with no toilet available.)
- Commonly used protections include the use of tampons or the cup.
- Every female diver is aware of how she feels during each stage of her menstrual cycle and can assess her own ability to dive at that time. In general, there is no proven increased risk for a menstruating woman to dive.

## PREGNANCY

There has been a long and hard debate about the safety of diving during pregnancy.

There are some known factors but most concerns are theoretical:

- Nausea and vomiting commonly occur, especially during the first trimester.
- The distended abdomen and enlargement of breasts can be a problem when fitting weight belts and wetsuits.
- The abdominal contents may be injured when clambering over the side of small boats.
- The growing uterus will restrict respiratory function, especially in the third trimester and may limit exercise tolerance.
- High partial pressures of oxygen, nitrogen and carbon dioxide could have toxic or teratogenic effects on the foetus.
- Venous bubbles bypassing the foetal pulmonary circulation through the foramen ovale could cause arterial gas embolism in the foetus.
- The foetus could have an increased susceptibility to decompression illness. Bubble formation in foetal tissue could have a teratogenic effect.
- Increased fluid retention during the second trimester onwards could interfere with Eustachian tube function.
- Increased fluid retention could predispose to maternal decompression illness.
- A UK study on scuba diving and pregnancy in 2006 could not find sufficient numbers of pregnant women diving to make any significant correlation between diving and foetal abnormalities (St Ledger Dowser).

**The general recommendation of all diving and medical organizations is not to dive during pregnancy or when trying to fall pregnant.**

## POST NATAL

- Adequate time for the cervix to close and the endometrium to heal should be allowed before resuming diving. A six-week delay before diving has been suggested though many women do not feel emotionally prepared for several months after parturition.
- General conditioning may be reduced after pregnancy and a supervised exercise program may be advised to regain fitness before diving.

- Breastfeeding should not be affected by diving.

## SEXUAL INTERCOURSE

- Although it is not relevant specifically to diving the risks of having sexual intercourse in and underwater is a frequently asked question.
- The sea and freshwater lakes contain a variety of microorganisms, which will be encouraged to enter the vagina by sexual penetration and intercourse. The risk of the organisms entering the vagina will depend on the patency of the cervical canal, the consistency of the cervical mucus and the presence of an intrauterine device.
- Both pelvic infections and Bartholin's abscess have been reported following in-water sexual intercourse.
- Buoyancy control could be a problem and with poor breath control could predispose to barotrauma.
- Safe sex practices should not be forgotten.

## TAMPONS

- There have been isolated anecdotal reports of tampons causing discomfort during diving but none of them become impacted.
- Many women wear tampons whilst diving with no discomfort.

## URINARY INCONTINENCE

- More women in their fifties and sixties are learning to dive.
- Urinary incontinence, urge, stress or overflow, affects 10-25% of adult women. It is often socially disabling, whilst diving incontinence may be aggravated by lifting heavy equipment and by immersion and cold diuresis.
- Many women deliberately reduce their fluid intake whilst outdoors to try to reduce their dependency on toilet facilities and avoid incontinence. This may predispose to decompression illness (DCI).
- Alpha-agonists such as pseudoephedrine (Sudafed) have been used for the treatment of stress incontinence. The bladder neck and proximal urethra have abundant alpha receptors. Activation of these receptors by alpha-agonists leads to an increase in smooth muscle tone.

## FURTHER READING:


1. Cameron-Strange A. Female Urinary Incontinence. Current Therapeutics 1999 Feb: 19-24
2. Klien S, Spiegel M, Engelhardt K, Schmidauer C, Ulmer H, Diepers M, Mutzbauer T, Schmutzhard E. Menstrual cycle-dependent right-to-left shunting: A single-blinded transcranial Doppler sonography study.
3. Morales M, Dumps P, Extermann P. Pregnancy and scuba diving: what precautions? J Gynecol Obstet Biol Reprod 1999; 28(2): 118-23
4. St Leger Dowse M, Bryson P, Gunby A, Fife W. Men and Women in Diving. The Diving Diseases Research Centre, Fort Bovisand, Plymouth, Devon, UK. 1994.
5. St. Leger Dowse M, Bryson P, Gunby A, Fife W. Scuba diving and the menstrual cycle: interim data from the second year of a four year prospective study of diving women. SPUMS J 1999; 29(1): 50-53
6. St Leger Dowse M, Gunby A, Moncad R, Fife C, Bryson P. Scuba diving and pregnancy: can we determine safe limits? J Obstet Gynaecol. 2006; 26: 509-13.
7. St Leger Dowse M, Gunby A, Phil D, Moncad R, Fife C, Morsman J, Bryson P. Problems associated with scuba diving are not evenly distributed across a menstrual cycle. J Obstet Gynaecol. 2006; 26: 216-21.
8. Uguccioni D M, Moon R, Taylor M. DAN explore fitness and diving issues for women. Alert Diver 1999 Jan/ Feb: 41-44

# Appendices 23

## EQUALISING THE EARS

## POINTS TO PONDER

- Barotrauma to the middle ear is the most common injury sustained by divers because the middle ear is the only air cavity in the body which needs active equalization whilst diving. Air must travel from the nasopharynx through the Eustachian tube into the middle ear cavity to equalize the pressure across the tympanic membrane.
- Normally the eustachian tube opens on average every second swallow. One swallows about once a minute whilst awake and once every five minutes whilst asleep. Swallowing does not automatically occur whilst mouth breathing, especially with a regulator in the mouth.
- During a dive equalization of the middle ear may become difficult due to:
  - » Venous congestion of the sub-mucosal veins from head-down positions encountered during diving.
  - » Congestion of the nasal mucosa from breathing cold air causes reflex vasodilation of the sub-mucosal venous sinuses.
  - » Mucous plugs blocking the Eustachian tubes, caused by breathing dry air, and reduced swallowing cause the nasal mucus to become more viscous.
  - » The soft tissues in the nasopharynx are distorted by gravity when in a head-down position.

For these reasons, it is important to descend feet first. Tolerance to pressure changes may be influenced by:

- The amount of air in the mastoid sinuses. Individuals with a large mastoid sinus volume will be less tolerant to pressure change.
- Distensibility of the tympanic membrane (TM). If the TM is very distensible it will more readily be able to accommodate volume changes within the middle ear without discomfort.
- Ease of equalization may be influenced by:
  - » The patency of the Eustachian tube is highly variable between individuals.
  - » Mechanical obstruction e.g., polyps.
  - » Secretions in the nasopharynx are increased by smoking.
  - » Mucosal oedema in the nasopharynx is caused by allergy or infection.

- Most problems are caused by poor understanding and technique. It is advisable to practice middle ear equalization on land until it becomes easy. Moreover, inflating the middle ears before submerging will give a pillow of air behind the TM and aid further equalizations on the descent.

There are several techniques described to open the Eustachian tubes:

## Valsalva Manoeuvre (Antonio-Maria Valsalva)

- Simply pinch the nostrils closed, close the mouth and exhale gently into the nose to raise the pressure in the nasopharynx. If it does not work then the pressure can quickly be increased but it has been suggested not to continue the pressure for more than 5 seconds (Roydhouse).
- Techniques that may help the manoeuvres include wiggling the jaw, laterally flexing the neck or swallowing.
- If the exhalation is too severe or prolonged, the eustachian tube can be locked closed preventing equalization. Excessive force can rarely cause vitreous haemorrhage and orbital hematoma (Katz), (Taylor).
- If the Valsalva manoeuvres are prolonged or very forceful the CSF pressure can rise and be transmitted through the aqueduct of the cochlea into the inner ear, where the round window can be distended and even ruptured.

## Toynbee technique (Joseph Toynbee)

- Simply pinch the nostrils closed and swallow.

## Edmonds technique (Carl Edmonds)

- While tensing the soft palate (the soft tissue at the back of the roof of your mouth) and throat muscles and pushing the jaw forward and down, do a Valsalva manoeuvre.

## Lowry technique

- A combination of Valsalva and Toynbee, while keeping the nostrils closed, blow and swallow concurrently.

## Frenzel Manoeuvre (Herman Frenzel)

- Close the mouth, nose and glottis (as if about to lift a heavy weight). Pinch the nostrils closed then force the base of the tongue and the palate against the posterior wall of the nasopharynx (as if starting to say the letter "K" or guttural "guh" sound). The effort is very brief and can be quickly repeated several times.
- This manoeuvre will inflate the eustachian tube without using the pressure effects of the lungs so being independent of breathing.
- Voluntary Tube Opening (Béance Tubaire Volontaire)
- A controlled contraction of the soft palate and of the upper throat muscles to overcome the normal elasticity of the eustachian tube, holding the tube open for equalization of pressure.
- First described by French divers and was commonly known as "beance tubaire voluntaire" or BTV. The technique is commonly used by experienced divers who seem to learn the technique automatically.

## FURTHER READING:

1. Jones W L. Valsalva Manoeuvre induced vitreous haemorrhage. J Am Optometric Assoc 1995; 66(5):301-4
2. Katz B, Carmody B. Subperiosteal orbital haematoma induced by the Valsalva manoeuvre. Am J Ophthalmol 1985; 100: 617 Roydhouse N. The Valsalva Manoeuvre (letter). SPUMS J 1996; 26(3): 171
3. Roydhouse N. Underwater Ear and Nose Care. Best Books. 1993.
4. Taylor D. The Valsalva Manoeuvre: a critical review. SPUMS J 1996; 26(1): 8-13

## INTERPRETATION OF PULMONARY FUCTION TESTING

- Simple respiratory function testing has always been accepted as an essential part of the diving medical to try and identify asymptomatic yet significant lung disease.
- Respiratory function testing is only as good as the extent of subject cooperation, the equipment used, the training and skill of the operator and the experience of the reporter. Of those indices, FVC, FEV1 and FVC/FEV1 ratio, easily measured by simple spirometric equipment, the FEV1/FVC ratio has the smallest range of normal variation and is the most specific for identifying obstructive airway disease. Usually, about 75% of normal-sized vital capacity is expelled in a second.
- People with restrictive lung disease will have a low FVC so their FEV1/FVC ratio will be increased and may even be 100%.
- If a diver, especially if they are tall, an elite athlete or a swimmer has a large vital capacity e.g., 130% of predicted, but a normal FEV1, 100% of predicted, it will result in a low FEV1/FVC ratio. Such a diver is in no danger of pulmonary barotrauma through small airway closure.
- In a review of cases of pulmonary barotrauma in navy personnel training for submarine escape a reduced FVC was the only simple spirometric measurement that had any predictive value for pulmonary barotrauma and arterial gas embolism.
- An individual should be considered fit to dive when the main spirometric parameters (FVC, FEV1, FEV1/FVC) are within 90% of the confidence interval (CI) (viz: Z-score of ± 1.64) and there are no signs of pathology in the history or physical examination. If a person's PFT is outside the 95% CI (Z-score ± 1.96), further assessment is advised (Wingelaar).

We recommend that all doctors doing dive medicals have a computerized spirometer that prints out all measurements alongside predicted values. Any diver who has FVC or FEV1 below 80% or an FEV1/FVC ratio below 90% should be reviewed and further evaluated. If there is still doubt then referral to a respiratory physician is recommended.

The use of spirometry should follow internationally accepted standards of standardisation, such as the Standardization of Spirometry 2019 Update; an Official American Thoracic Society and European Respiratory Society Technical Statement (available at: https://www.atsjournals.org/doi/10.1164/rccm.201908-1590ST)

## FURTHER READING:


1. Bates D V. Respiratory function in disease. 3rd ed Philadelphia: WB Saunders; 1989
2. Benton P J, Francis T J R, Pethybridge R J. Spirometric indices and the risk of pulmonary barotrauma in submarine escape training. Undersea Hyper Med 1999; 26 (4): 213-217
3. Pain M C. Basic tests of respiratory function. Australian Prescriber 2000; 23(1): 10-12
4. Pierce R, Johns D P. Spirometry: the measurement and interpretation of ventilatory function in clinical practice. Melbourne; National Asthma Campaign; 1995
5. Wingelaar TT, Clarijs P, van Ooij PJAM, Koch DAA, van Hulst RA. Modern assessment of pulmonary function in divers cannot rely on old reference values. Diving and Hyperbaric Medicine. 2018 March;48(1):17–22. doi:10.28920/dhm48.1.17-22. PMID: 29557097.
6. Wingelaar TT, Clarijs P, van Ooij PJAM, Koch DAA, van Hulst RA. The lower limit for FEV1/FVC in dive medical assessments: a retrospective study. Diving Hyperb Me. 2021 Dec 20;51(4):368-372. doi: 10.28920/dhm51.4.368-372. PMID: 34897602, PMCID: PMC8920896

# MEDICAL QUESTIONNAIRES FOR FITNESS TO DIVE ASSESSMENT

# THE SOUTH PACIFIC UNDERWATER MEDICINE SOCIETY

SPUMS

# GUIDELINES ON MEDICAL RISK ASSESSMENT FOR RECREATIONAL DIVING

# SECTION B

# SUGGESTED SCOPE OF A MEDICAL QUESTIONNAIRE FOR SCREENING CANDIDATES FOR RECREATIONAL SCUBA DIVING

# HEALTH STATEMENT FOR PERSONS WISHING TO UNDERTAKE SCUBA-DIVING TRAINING

The provision of inaccurate, incomplete or misleading information, or withholding any information is likely to place you at risk and renders any subsequent medical opinion unreliable.

## Introduction

This is a medical questionnaire designed to identify any health issues that may increase the risk to you from undertaking SCUBA diving.

In order to undertake dive training you will be required to sign this form on the understanding that relevant medical details may be passed to your dive trainer.

You will also be informed of some potential risks involved in scuba diving and of the conduct required of you during the scuba training programme. Your signature on this statement is required for you to participate in the scuba training program offered.

If you are under 18 years of age, you must have this questionnaire signed by a parent or guardian.

Training to be offered by________________________________________and

____________________________________ (Instructors) located at (Facility)

____________________________________________________________

____________________________________________________________

Diving is an exciting and demanding activity. When performed correctly, applying correct techniques, it is relatively safe. To scuba dive safely, you should not be extremely overweight or out of condition. Diving can be strenuous under certain conditions. Your lungs, heart and circulation must be in good health. All body air spaces such as the sinuses and middle ears must be normal and healthy. A person with heart disease, a current head cold or lung congestion, epilepsy (fits), any severe medical problem or who is under the influence of alcohol or drugs should not dive. If you have asthma, heart disease, other chronic medical conditions or you are taking medications on a regular basis, you should inform the doctor and the instructor before participating in this programme.

You will also learn from the instructor the important safety rules regarding breathing and ear clearing while scuba diving. Improper use of scuba equipment can result in serious injury. You must be thoroughly instructed in its use under direct supervision of a qualified instructor to use it safely.

If you have any additional questions regarding this Medical Statement or the Medical Questionnaire section, review them with your instructor before signing.

**Candidate initials**__________________

**Please read carefully before signing.**

1. Surname ______________________ Other Names ___________________________

2. Date of Birth (dd/mm/yyyy) _____________________

3. Address _________________________________________________

_________________________________________________

State: Postcode _________________________________________________

4. Sex Male / Female

5. Telephone (Home) ____________________

6. Principal Occupation _____________________

7. Telephone (Work) ____________________

8. Email (Optional) _____________________

9. How often do you exercise (minutes per week)? _

What is your estimated level of intensity of that exercise (High-Medium-Low)?

____________________________________________________________

10. Are you taking any prescription tablets, medicines or drugs?

List: ______________________________________________

______________________________________________

11. Have you had any reactions to drugs or medicines or foods?

Details: ______________________________________________

12. Tobacco Smoking History.

Do you smoke tobacco now? Y/N

Have you ever smoked tobacco? Y/N

How many cigarettes per day do/did you smoke and for how many years?

______________________________________________________

If other forms of tobacco, please detail__________________________

13. Do you drink alcohol?______________________________________Y/N

Estimate how many standard drinks per night or week.____________________

______________________________________________________________

14. Do you currently consume illicit drugs? Y/N

Detail:______________________________________________________

**Please answer the following questions on your past or present medical history (from question 15 onwards) with a YES or NO.**

- If you have never heard of the condition or had the diagnosis applied to you – then reply **NO**
- If you are not confident that you understand the question, then leave this blank and discuss with the doctor

| Have you ever had or do you now have any of the following? | YES | NO | Physician's comments |
|---|---|---|---|
| 15. Any continuing eye or visual problems (apart from needing glasses or contact lenses)? | | | |
| 16. Sinusitis (e.g. hay fever, sinus infections)? | | | |
| 17. Any other nose or throat problem (apart from previous coughs and colds)? | | | |
| 18. Dentures or plates that are removable? | | | |
| 19. Deafness or ringing noises in ear(s)? | | | |
| 20. Discharging ears or other infections? | | | |
| 21. Previous ear operation (including as a child)? | | | |
| 22. Giddiness or loss of balance? | | | |
| 23. Severe motion sickness? | | | |
| 24. Any ear problems or severe headaches when flying in aircraft? | | | |
| 25. Severe or frequent headaches, including migraine? | | | |
| 26. Faints or blackouts? | | | |
| 27. Convulsions, fits or epilepsy? | | | |
| 28. Any episodes of unconsciousness? | | | |
| 29. Depression requiring medical treatment? | | | |
| 30. Claustrophobia? | | | |
| 31. Mental illness or mental health issues requiring therapy of treatment? | | | |
| 32. Bronchitis or pneumonia? | | | |
| 33. Pleurisy or severe chest pain? | | | |
| 34. Coughing up phlegm or blood? | | | |

| Have you ever had or do you now have any of the following? | YES | NO | Physician's comments |
|---|---|---|---|
| 35. Chronic or persistent cough? | | | |
| 36. Tuberculosis ("TB")? | | | |
| 37. Pneumothorax ("collapsed lung")? | | | |
| 38. Frequent chest colds? | | | |
| 39. Asthma or wheezing? | | | |
| 40. Use a puffer (medication inhaler for asthma)? | | | |
| 41. Any other chest complaint? | | | |
| 42. Operation on chest, lungs, or heart? | | | |
| 43. Peptic ulcer or acid reflux requiring treatment? | | | |
| 44. Vomiting blood or passing red or black motions? | | | |
| 45. Jaundice, hepatitis or liver disease? | | | |
| 46. Malaria? | | | |
| 47. Severe loss of weight? | | | |
| 48. Hernia or rupture? | | | |
| 49. Major joint or back injury? | | | |
| 50. Paralysis, muscle weakness or numbness? | | | |
| 51. Kidney disease? | | | |
| 52. Diabetes? | | | |
| 53. Blood disease or bleeding problem? | | | |
| 54. Could you be pregnant, or are you trying to become pregnant? | | | |
| **CARDIOVASCULAR RISK QUESTIONS** | | | |
| 55. Do you have any known heart disease or have your ever consulted a cardiologist (specialist heart doctor)? | | | |
| 56. Is there a family history of heart disease or diabetes? | | | |
| 57. Is there a family history of sudden death at a young age? | | | |
| 58. Are you ever aware of a racing or irregularly beating heart, or any other known problems with your heart beat? | | | |
| 59. Have you ever had giddiness, light headedness of periods of unconsciousness whether or not associated with exercise? | | | |
| 60. Do you ever get discomfort in your chest with exertion (angina)? | | | |
| 61. Do you ever get very short of breath on exertion (out of proportion to the exercise, or before your legs get tired)? | | | |
| 62. Have you ever been short of breath lying down or woken from sleep with breathlessness? | | | |

| CARDIOVASCULAR RISK QUESTIONS | YES | NO | Physician's comments |
|---|---|---|---|
| 63. Do you have a pacemaker or implanted defibrillator? | | | |
| 64. Have you ever had an operation on the heart including any placement of stents? | | | |
| 65. Have you ever failed or had a significant medical issue with a diving medical in the past? | | | |
| 66. Have you ever had a diagnosis of the following: | | | |
| • High blood pressure? | ____ | ____ | |
| • Rheumatic fever or problems with your heart valves? | ____ | ____ | |
| • High cholesterol? | ____ | ____ | |
| • Immersion pulmonary oedema? | ____ | ____ | |
| • Heart failure or a problem with heart muscle including cardiomyopathy or obstructive coronary heart disease? | ____ | ____ | |
| • A hole in the heart (PFO, ASD, VSD) or other congenital heart disease? | ____ | ____ | |
| • Blood clots on the lungs? | ____ | ____ | |
| • A stroke? | ____ | ____ | |

**Water skills and diving history**

Previous Diving Experience? When, and how many dives?

Details: ______________________________

______________________________

Previous qualifications (if any): ______________________________

Can you swim? ______________________________

Have you ever had any problem during or after swimming or diving?

Details: ______________________________

Have you ever had decompression illness?

Details: ______________________________

Do you snorkel dive regularly? ______________________________

## Candidate Statement

I certify that the above information is true and complete to the best of my knowledge. I hereby authorise (dive training organisation) ________________________ to pass this information to a diving doctor of my choosing. I also authorise that doctor to obtain or supply medical information regarding me to other doctors as may be necessary for medical purposes in my personal interest.

**Signed:** ______________________________________ **Date:** ____________________

**Note**
Any chronic disease, such as hepatitis A, B, C, AIDS or tuberculosis, may increase your risks from diving. If you have a chronic disease please discuss it with the doctor who will then be able to advise you whether you will be at increased risk.

## SPUMS PRE-DIVE MEDICAL FORM FOR ENTRY-LEVEL SCUBA DIVERS

**Append the diver medical statement above**

**Notes or additions to medical history:** ______________________________

______________________________

______________________________

## MEDICAL EXAMINATION: To be completed by an Approved Medical Practitioner

| 1. Height<br>cm | 2. Weight<br>kg | 3.Visual acuity<br>R 6/ Corrected 6/<br>L 6/ Corrected 6/ | 4. Blood Pressure<br>mmHg | 5. Pulse rate<br>bpm |
|---|---|---|---|---|
| 6. Urinalysis<br>Albumin<br><br>Glucose | 7. Respiratory function tests including: (attach results)<br>FVC<br><br>$FEV_1$<br><br>Ratio (%) | | 8. CXR (if required)<br>Date:<br>Place:<br>Result: | |

| 9. Audiometry dB | (Hz) 500 | 1000 | 1500 | 2000 | 3000 | 4000 | 6000 | 8000 |
|---|---|---|---|---|---|---|---|---|
| Right | | | | | | | | |
| Left | | | | | | | | |
| 10. ECG (if indicated) | | | | | | | | |

| Clinical Examination/Assessment | Normal | Abnormal | Notes on any abnormalities |
|---|---|---|---|
| 11. Nose, septum, airway | | | |
| 12. Mouth, throat, teeth, bite | | | |
| 13. External auditory canal | | | |
| 14. Tympanic membrane | | | |
| 15. Middle ear autoinflation | | | |
| 16. Neurological<br>Eye movements<br>Pupillary reflexes<br>Limb reflexes<br>Finger-nose<br>Sharpened Romberg Test | | | |
| 17. Abdomen | | | |
| 18. Chest auscultation | | | |
| 19. Cardiac auscultation | | | |
| 20. Other abnormalities | | | |

**STATEMENT OF HEALTH FOR RECREATIONAL DIVING**

***This Section to be completed by a Medical Practitioner with appropriate training in diving medicine***

This is to certify that I have today interviewed and examined:

Name.......................................................................................................................................

Address...................................................................................................................................

..................................................................................................................................................

Date of birth................./................./................

***Initial the statements that apply:***

| | |
|---|---|
| | I have assessed the candidate in accordance with the SPUMS Recreational Dive Medical. |
| | I can find no conditions which are incompatible with compressed gas, scuba and surface supplied breathing apparatus (SSBA) and / or breath-hold diving. |
| | I have explained the health risks of diving disclosed by this examination to the candidate and we have discussed how these risks may be reduced. The candidate appears to have a good understanding of these risks. |
| | Based upon my assessment, the candidate should not dive with compressed gases (scuba and SSBA). |
| | Based upon my assessment, the candidate should not breath-hold dive. |

Advice: (append further notes as required)

Condition 1: ___________________________

Condition 2: ___________________________

.................................................................. ........../........../..........

(Signature of Medical Practitioner) (Date)

(Name, address and telephone number of the Medical Practitioner)

***This Section to be completed by the Candidate***

***Initial the statements that apply:***

........... I understand the health risks that I may encounter in diving and how these risks may be reduced.

........... I also understand that the medical practitioner's recommendation herewith is based, in part, upon the disclosure of my medical history.

........... I agree to accept any responsibility and liability for health risks associated with my participation in underwater diving, including those that are due to or are influenced by a change in my health and / or my failure to disclose any existing or past health condition to the medical practitioner.

........... I hereby authorise the medical practitioner to supply information with regard to my medical fitness to dive to the diving instructor.

.................................................................. .................................................................. ...../...../........

Signature of candidate Name of Candidate Date

## Pro-forma statement to be added to the certificate in Section B, for use when counselling divers with diabetes about their diving

## STATEMENT REGARDING DIABETES AND DIVING

I, ................................................ hereby acknowledge my understanding and acceptance of the following issues:

1. Altered consciousness, heart attack, or exhaustion during diving may lead to drowning and other life-threatening complications.
2. A history of diabetes implies a greater risk of these events.

<u>Moreover,</u>

3. Diving itself may make these events more likely in a diabetic diver by precipitating hypoglycaemia, or imposing high physical demands in certain situations.

<u>And</u>

4. That because of the issues described at 1 – 3, people with diabetes are frequently considered unfit to dive.

<u>However, I also understand</u>

5. That the extra risk in diving for a diabetic diver who meets certain criteria for selection as a diver and who practices appropriate diabetic diving technique is likely to be relatively small. Unfortunately, this risk has not been quantified.
6. That any decision for a person with diabetes to dive must be based on the perceived benefit weighed against the potential risk.

<u>Having decided to proceed with diver training, I acknowledge</u>

7. That Dr ........................................'s assessment of my risk in diving has been based in part on my own reports of blood glucose control, and my general state of health. I acknowledge my responsibility for the accuracy of those reports.
8. That if the pattern of my diabetes changes significantly, or if I suffer any adverse diabetes-related event in which I require assistance or medical consultation at any time, then the risk of diving may be increased and I should cease diving and discuss the issue with Dr.......................................... again.
9. That I should not dive during any period likely to be associated with worsening of my glycaemic control, such as during a cold or other illness.
10. That if I find diving precipitates any problems in relation to my diabetes, I should cease diving forthwith and seek review with Dr ..................................................
11. That I understand the necessity to more closely monitor and adjust my glucose levels on diving days, in accordance with the diabetic diving guidelines.
12. That I have read, understood, and had an opportunity to ask questions about the diabetic diving guidelines.
13. That I understand the necessity to inform my dive buddy and dive group about my diabetes.
14. That I must undergo annual review with Dr.............................................................. or another diving doctor as long as I continue to dive.

<u>Finally, I understand that</u>

15. being informed of the above issues, having had my questions answered, and having been counselled about my risk in diving, I accept that I am responsible for my decision to dive. I hold no one else responsible for any adverse consequences of this decision.

Signed:..........................................................................Date:................................

# DIVE MEDICAL | PARTICIPANT QUESTIONNAIRE

Recreational scuba diving and freediving require good physical and mental health. There are a few medical conditions which can be hazardous while diving, listed below. Those who have, or are predisposed to, any of these conditions, should be evaluated by a physician. This Diver Medical Participant Questionnaire provides a basis to determine if you should seek out that evaluation. If you have any concerns about your diving fitness not represented on this form, consult with your physician before diving. If you are feeling ill, avoid diving. If you think you may have a contagious disease, protect yourself and others by not participating in dive training and/ or dive activities. References to "diving" in this form encompass both recreational scuba diving and freediving. This form is principally designed as an initial medical screen for new divers but is also appropriate for divers taking continuing education. For your safety, and that of others who may dive with you, answer all questions honestly.

**Directions**

**Complete this questionnaire as a prerequisite to a recreational scuba diving or freediving course. Note to women:** If you are pregnant, or attempting to become pregnant, *do not dive.*

| | | | |
|---|---|---|---|
| 1 | I have had problems with my lungs, breathing, heart and/or blood affecting my normal physical or mental performance. | Yes<br>Go to box A | No ☐ |
| 2 | I am over 45 years of age. | Yes<br>Go to box B | No ☐ |
| 3 | I struggle to perform moderate exercise (for example, walk 1.6 kilometre/one mile in 14 minutes or swim 200 meters/yards without resting), OR I have been unable to participate in a normal physical activity due to fitness or health reasons within the past 12 months. | Yes ☐ * | No ☐ |
| 4 | I have had problems with my eyes, ears, or nasal passages/sinuses. | Yes<br>Go to box C | No ☐ |
| 5 | I have had surgery within the last 12 months, OR I have ongoing problems related to past surgery. | Yes ☐* | No ☐ |
| 6 | I have lost consciousness, had migraine headaches, seizures, stroke, significant head injury, or suffer from persistent neurologic injury or disease. | Yes<br>Go to box D | No ☐ |
| 7 | I am currently undergoing treatment (or have required treatment within the last five years) for psychological problems, personality disorder, panic attacks, or an addiction to drugs or alcohol; or, I have been diagnosed with a learning or developmental disability. | Yes<br>Go to box E | No ☐ |
| 8 | I have had back problems, hernia, ulcers, or diabetes. | Yes<br>Go to box F | No ☐ |
| 9 | I have had stomach or intestine problems, including recent diarrhoea. | Yes<br>Go to box G | No ☐ |
| 10 | I am taking prescription medications (with the exception of birth control or anti-malarial drugs other than mefloquine (Lariam). | Yes ☐ * | No ☐ |

**Participant Signature**

**If you answered NO** to all 10 questions above, a medical evaluation is not required. Please read and agree to the participant statement below by signing and dating it.

**Participant Statement:** I have answered all questions honestly, and understand that I accept responsibility for any consequences resulting from any questions I may have answered inaccurately or for my failure to disclose any existing or past health conditions.

Participant Signature (or, if a minor, participant's parent/guardian signature required. ____________________

Date (dd/mm/yyyy) ____________________

Participant Name (Print) ____________________

Birthdate (dd/mm/yyyy) ____________________

Instructor Name (Print) ____________________

Facility Name (Print) ____________________

*** If you answered YES** to questions 3, 5 or 10 above **OR** to any of the questions on page 2, please read and agree to the statement above by signing and dating it **AND take all three pages of this form (Participant Questionnaire and the Physician's Evaluation Form)** to your physician for a medical evaluation. Participation in a diving course requires your physician's approval.

## DIVER MEDICAL | PARTICIPANT QUESTIONNAIRE CONTINUED

| BOX A – I HAVE/HAVE HAD: | | |
|---|---|---|
| Chest surgery, heart surgery, heart valve surgery, an implantable medical device (eg., stent, pacemaker, neurostimulator), pneumothorax, and/or chronic lung disease. | Yes* | No ☐ |
| Asthma, wheezing, severe allergies, hay fever or congested airways within the last 12 months that limits my physical activity/exercise. | Yes* | No ☐ |
| A problem or illness involving my heart such as: angina, chest pain on exertion, heart failure, immersion pulmonary oedema, heart attack or stroke, OR am taking medication for any heart condition. | Yes* | No ☐ |
| Recurrent bronchitis and currently coughing within the past 12 months, OR have been diagnosed with emphysema. | Yes* | No ☐ |
| Symptoms affecting my lungs, breathing, heart and/or blood in the last 30 days that impair my physical or mental performance. | Yes* | No ☐ |
| **BOX B – I AM OVER 45 YEARS OF AGE AND:** | | |
| I currently smoke or inhale nicotine by other means. | Yes* | No ☐ |
| I have a high cholesterol level. | Yes* | No ☐ |

| | | |
|---|---|---|
| I have high blood pressure. | Yes* | No ☐ |
| I have had a close blood relative die suddenly or of cardiac disease or stroke before the age of 50, OR have a family history of heart disease before age 50 (including abnormal heart rhythms, coronary artery disease or cardiomyopathy). | Yes* | No ☐ |
| BOX C – I HAVE/HAVE HAD: | | |
| Sinus surgery within the last 6 months. | Yes* | No ☐ |
| Ear disease or ear surgery, hearing loss, or problems with balance. | Yes* | No ☐ |
| Recurrent sinusitis within the past 12 months. | Yes* | No ☐ |
| Eye surgery within the past 3 months. | Yes* | No ☐ |
| BOX D – I HAVE/HAVE HAD: | | |
| Head injury with loss of consciousness within the past 5 years. | Yes* | No ☐ |
| Persistent neurologic injury or disease. | Yes* | No ☐ |
| Recurring migraine headaches within the past 12 months, or take medications to prevent them. | Yes* | No ☐ |
| Blackouts or fainting (full/partial loss of consciousness) within the last 5 years. | Yes* | No ☐ |
| Epilepsy, seizures, or convulsions, OR take medications to prevent them. | Yes* | No ☐ |
| BOX E – I HAVE/HAVE HAD: | | |
| Behavioural health, mental or psychological problems requiring medical/psychiatric treatment. | Yes* | No ☐ |
| Major depression, suicidal ideation, panic attacks, uncontrolled bipolar disorder requiring medication/psychiatric treatment. | Yes* | No ☐ |
| Been diagnosed with a mental health condition or a learning/developmental disorder that requires ongoing care or special accommodation. | Yes* | No ☐ |
| An addiction to drugs or alcohol requiring treatment within the last 5 years. | Yes* | No ☐ |
| BOX F – I HAVE/HAVE HAD: | | |
| Recurrent back problems in the last 6 months that limit my everyday activity. | Yes* | No ☐ |
| Back or spinal surgery within the last 12 months. | Yes* | No ☐ |
| Diabetes, either drug or diet controlled, OR gestational diabetes within the last 12 months. | Yes* | No ☐ |
| An uncorrected hernia that limits my physical abilities. | Yes* | No ☐ |
| Active or untreated ulcers, problem wounds, or ulcer surgery within the last 6 months. | Yes* | No ☐ |
| BOX G – I HAVE HAD: | | |
| Ostomy surgery and do not have medical clearance to swim or engage in physical activity. | Yes* | No ☐ |

| | | |
|---|---|---|
| Dehydration requiring medical intervention within the last 7 days. | Yes* | No ☐ |
| Active or untreated stomach or intestinal ulcers or ulcer surgery within the last 6 months. | Yes* | No ☐ |
| Frequent heartburn, regurgitation, or gastroesophageal reflux disease (GERD). | Yes* | No ☐ |
| Active or uncontrolled ulcerative colitis or Crohn's disease. | Yes* | No ☐ |
| Bariatric surgery within the last 12 months. | Yes* | No ☐ |

*Physician's medical evaluation required (see page 1). 

## DIVER MEDICAL | MEDICAL EXAMINER'S EVALUATION FORM

**Participant Name** **Birthdate**

______________________________ ______________

(Print) Date (dd/mm/yyyy)

The above-named person requests your opinion of his/her medical suitability to participate in recreational scuba diving or freediving training or activity. Please visit uhms.org for medical guidance on medical conditions as they relate to diving. Review the areas relevant to your patient as part of your evaluation.

## Evaluation Result

☐ Approved – I find no conditions that I consider incompatible with recreational scuba diving or freediving.

☐ Not approved – I find conditions that I consider incompatible with recreational scuba diving or freediving.

______________________________ ______________

Signature of certified medical doctor or other legally certified medical provider Date (dd/mm/yyyy)

**Medical Examiner's Name** ______________________________

# Glossary

**Alveolitis:** inflammation of alveoli.

**Alveolus:** pl alveoli: an air sac of the lungs.

**Ambient pressure:** the surrounding pressure.

**Aminoglycoside:** an antibiotic containing amino sugars linked by glycoside. An important adverse effect is nerve deafness.

**Aneurysm:** A circumscribed sac-like bulging of a blood vessel, usually an artery.

**Angina:** a constricting pain in the chest due to insufficient blood supply to the heart.

**Angiogram:** X-ray of a blood vessel obtained by outlining the structure with a radio-opaque material.

**Angioplasty:** surgical reconstruction of a blood vessel.

**Anticholinergic:** inhibiting the action of a parasympathetic nerve.

**Apex, pl apices:** the tip or pointed end of a conical structure, such as the heart or lung.

**Aplasia:** complete or partial failure of a tissue to develop.

**Arterial gas embolism (AGE):** the medical condition caused by bubbles of air, usually in diving from an over-distended ruptured lung when the bubbles enter the pulmonary circulation and travel to the arterial circulation where they block the arteries.

**Arteritis:** inflammation of an artery.

**Arthralgia:** pain in a joint.

**Asthenia:** loss of strength; weakness.

**Ataxia:** lack of muscular coordination.

**Atelectasis:** a shrunken and airless state of the lung or part of it due to failure of expansion or resorption of air from the alveoli.

**Athetosis:** a condition marked by constant, slow, involuntary writhing movements of the hands, fingers and sometimes the feet.

**Atlantoaxial:** relating to the atlas and axis; as the articulation between C1 and C2 vertebrae.

**Atmosphere absolute (ATA):** the atmospheric pressure at sea level.

**Atony:** lack of normal tone.

**Atopy:** denoting an allergy characteristic of humans and tending to be inherited eg. hay fever and asthma.

**Avascular necrosis:** death of tissue in a circumscribed area due to loss of blood supply.

**Axon:** the long cytoplasmic process of a nerve cell which combines to form a nerve.

**Barotrauma:** any disease or injury due to unequal pressures between an air space within the body and the ambient pressure.

**Bleb:** an abnormal pocket of air in the lungs.

**Bradycardia:** an abnormal slowness of the heartbeat.

**Bronchospasm:** spasmodic constriction of the bronchial tubes.

**Bruit:** abnormal sound heard over a narrowed artery as the blood is pushed through.

**Bulla:** an abnormal pocket of air in the lungs.

**Burr hole:** a hole made through the skull.

**Caries:** localized, progressive decay of teeth.

**Cerebral vascular disease:** diseased and often narrowed arteries supplying the brain.

**Chemosis:** an eye disorder marked by swelling of the conjunctiva around the cornea.

**Claudication:** pain in the legs caused by the narrowing of arteries reducing the blood supply to the leg's muscles.

**Cognition:** the intellectual process by which knowledge is acquired as opposed to emotional processes.

**Contusion:** a superficial injury or bruise.

**Decompression:** a change from one pressure to a lower pressure.

**Decompression dive:** a dive in which the diver is required to perform a decompression stop on returning to the surface defined by the decompression tables to prevent decompression illness.

**Decompression stop:** as the diver ascends they will stop at a specified depth for a specified time to allow off-gassing.

**Decompression illness (DCI):** a term to encompass all bubble-related problems arising from decompression, including decompression sickness and arterial gas embolism.

**Degeneration:** the deterioration of tissues with corresponding functional impairment as a result of injury or disease.

**Diplopia:** double vision.

**Dioptre:** the unit used to designate the refractive power of a lens or optical system.

**Diuresis:** discharge of increased amounts of urine.

**Diverticulum:** a saccular dilation protruding from the wall of a tubular organ.

**Drysuit:** a watertight garment that keeps the diver dry and under which they can wear clothing to keep them warm.

**Dysarthria:** impairment of the ability to produce clear speech.

**Dysrhythmia:** an irregularity of the heartbeat.

**Dystonia:** abnormal tone in muscles.

**Echocardiogram:** an outline of the structure of the heart produced by ultrasonic waves.

**Effusion:** the escape of body fluid into a body cavity.

**Emphysema:** swelling due to the abnormal pressure of air in tissues or cavities of the body.

**Encephalitis:** inflammation of the brain.

**Endometritis:** inflammation of the membranes lining the interior of the uterus.

**Endophthalmitis:** inflammation of the internal structures of the eye.

**Esophagitis:** inflammation of the oesophagus or gullet.

**Eustachian tube:** a muco-cartilaginous tube, about 1.5 cm long, connecting the back of the nose to the middle ear.

**Extrapyramidal:** outside of the pyramidal tracts.

**Fibrillation:** the rapid contraction or quivering of muscle fibrils, eg. of the atria or ventricles of the heart.

**Fibrosis:** the formation of fibrous tissue; denoting especially an abnormal degenerative process.

**First stage regulator:** a regulator attached to the scuba tank that reduces the tank pressure to an intermediate pressure that feeds the second stage regulator in the mouth.

**Fundoplication:** suturing of the fundus of the stomach.

**Gastrectomy:** surgical removal of part or all of the stomach.

**Gastrojejunostomy:** surgical creation of an opening between the stomach and jejunum.

**Haemolysis:** the liberation of haemoglobin from the red blood cells.

**Haematoma:** a localised mass of blood outside of the blood vessels.

**Haemodynamic:** of or relating to blood circulation.

**Haemothorax:** accumulation of blood between the lung and chest wall causing a collapse of the lung.

**Hemiplegia:** paralysis of one side of the body.

**Heterozygote:** a fertilized egg produced by the union of two gametes with different genetic compositions.

**Homozygote:** a fertilized egg produced by the union of two gametes with similar genetic composition.

**Hydrocephalus:** excessive accumulation in the ventricles of the brain or in the subarachnoid spaces.

**Hyperbaric chamber:** an air-tight chamber which can simulate the pressure at depth. It is used in the treatment of divers with decompression illness.

**Hypercapnia:** a higher-than-normal pCO2 level in the blood.

**Hyperglycaemia:** high blood glucose.

**Hypermetropia:** also, Hyperopia farsightedness: the rays of light entering the eye focus behind the retina.

**Hypertension:** high blood pressure.

**Hyperthermia:** a body temperature warmer than the normal 37°C/98.6°F.

**Hyperventilation:** over breathing to the extent that the pCO2 is reduced.

**Hyphaema:** a collection of blood in the anterior chamber of the eye.

**Hypochromic:** having less than the normal amount of pigment, eg. haemoglobin.

**Hypoglycaemia:** low blood glucose.

**Hypoplasia:** defective or incomplete development of an organ or a part.

**Hypotension:** low blood pressure.

**Hypothermia:** a body temperature lower than the normal 37°C/ 98.6°F.

**Hypoventilation:** under breathing to the extent that the pCO2 is elevated.

**Hypoxia:** lower than normal pO2 level in the blood.

**Idiopathic:** denoting a disease of unknown cause.

**Incarcerated:** confined; held fast, as an irreducible hernia.

**Infarct:** an area of necrosis in a tissue caused by an obstruction in the artery supplying the area.

**Insufficiency:** unable to perform a normal function.

**Intraocular:** within the eyeball.

**Ischemia:** lack of blood flow to an area of the body due to mechanical obstruction or functional constriction of a blood vessel.

**Keratitis:** inflammation of the cornea of the eye.

**Keratoconus:** a central conical protrusion of the cornea.

**Keratoplasty:** an operation in which the cornea or a portion of it is removed and replaced by healthy corneal tissue.

**Lacrimal caruncle:** a small reddish protuberance at the inner junction of the eyelids.

**Lacrimal punctum:** the minute opening of the lacrimal duct on the margin of each eyelid at the inner canthus.

**Lateral epicondylitis:** pain and tenderness of the tendons near the lateral epicondyle of the humerus.

**Lordosis:** abnormally increased forward curvature of the lumbar spine.

**Lymphadenopathy:** enlarged lymph nodes.

**Meatus:** a body channel or its opening.

**Mediastinum:** the central space in the chest between the lungs.

**Meningitis:** inflammation of the lining of the spinal cord and brain.

**Mesothelioma:** a malignant tumour of the pleura associated with exposure to asbestosis.

**Microcytosis:** a condition in which the red blood cells are smaller than normal.

**Middle ear:** air containing space in the ear behind the eardrum and connected to the back of the nose via the eustachian tube.

**Mitral valve:** the valve between the left atrium and ventricle of the heart.

**Mixed gas:** any mixture of gases used for breathing underwater that is not air, e.g., enriched air or Nitrox.

**Mononeuritis:** inflammation or degeneration of a single nerve trunk.

**Murmur:** a noise produced by the turbulent flow of blood through the heart.

**Myelopathy:** any disease of the spinal cord.

**Myocardial infarction:** deterioration and/or death of a portion of the heart muscle as a result of deprivation of its blood supply.

**Myocardium:** the middle and thickest layer of the heart wall composed of specialized striated muscle cells and intervening connective tissue.

**Myopathy:** any disease of muscular tissue.

**Myopia:** nearsightedness, light rays entering the eyeball focus in front of the retina.

**Myotonia:** temporary rigidity of a muscle or group of muscles.

**Nasolacrimal:** relating to the nose and structures producing and conveying tears.

**Nasopharynx:** the uppermost part of the pharynx, located above the level of the soft palate immediately behind the nasal cavity.

**Neuritis:** inflammation or degeneration of a nerve.

**Neuropathy:** any disease of the nervous system.

**Nystagmus:** an involuntary movement of the eyes in a horizontal, vertical or rotary direction.

**Ossicular chain:** the three bones of the middle ear; malleus, incus and stapes which together form a bony chain.

**Osteomyelitis:** infection of the bone.

**Otitis:** inflammation or infection of any part of the ear.

**Otorrhea:** discharge from the ear.

**Palpebral:** of or relating to the eyelids.

**Pancreatitis:** inflammation of the pancreas.

**Pancytopenia:** reduction of all the blood cell components of the blood.

**Paraesthesia:** an abnormal sensation, such as burning, tingling or numbness.

**Paradoxical arterial gas embolism:** gas bubbles moving from the right circulation to the left circulation, against normal pressure gradients or through pulmonary arteriovenous shunts.

**Paraphasias:** slight or partial weakness of both lower limbs.

**Parenchymal:** the characteristic tissue of an organ or gland, as distinguished from connective tissue.

**Partial pressure:** pressure exerted by a single component of a gas within a gas mixture, or dissolved in a liquid.

**Pericarditis:** inflammation of the pericardium, a sac that encloses the heart.

**Periosteum:** a thick fibrous membrane covering the surface of bones.

**Peripheral neuropathy:** inflammation of the nerves outside the central nervous system, especially in the limbs.

**Peripheral vascular disease:** diseased and often narrowed arteries in the outer body, away from the major organs, commonly seen in the aorta and arteries in the legs.

**Peritoneum:** the serous membrane lining the abdominal and pelvic cavities.

**Petechia:** a small haemorrhage appearing as a flat, purplish-red spot.

**Phacoemulsification:** removal of the lens of the eye afflicted with a cataract by means of a low-frequency ultrasonic needle.

**Photosensitivity:** hypersensitization of skin to sunlight or ultraviolet rays.

**Pneumocephalus:** air in the skull.

**Pneumomediastinum:** an abnormal collection of air between the lungs.

**Pneumonitis:** inflammation of the lungs.

**Pneumothorax:** an abnormal collection of air between the lung and the chest wall causing a collapse of the lung.

**Polyneuropathy:** a disease in which several peripheral nerves are affected at the same time.

**Presbyopia:** diminution of accommodation power in the eyes due to advancing age.

**Squeeze:** pain in the air spaces of the body caused by higher external pressure.

**Stenosis:** abnormal constriction of a blood vessel, heart valve, channel or orifice.

**Stomatitis:** inflammation of the mucous membrane of the mouth.

**Stridor:** a harsh, shrill respiratory sound.

**Surface interval:** the time between surfacing from one dive to descending on the next dive.

**Syncope:** a brief loss of consciousness; a faint.

**Tachycardia:** an abnormally fast heartbeat.

**Thermocline:** the intersection between two layers of water that are of distinctly different temperatures, the colder layer being the deeper.

**Thoracoplasty:** plastic surgery or repair of defects of the chest.

**Thrombocytopenia:** an abnormally low number of platelets in the blood.

**Thrombosis:** the formation or presence of a blood clot.

**Transudate:** a fluid that passes through a membrane, such as a capillary wall, as a result of differences in hydrostatic pressure.

**Tricuspid valve:** the valve between the right atrium and ventricle of the heart.

**Tuberculous:** afflicted with tuberculosis.

**Urticaria:** the eruption of transitory itchy wheals on the skin; hives.

**Valsalva manoeuvre:** a method of equalising the middle ear. See page 153.

**Pressure:** any force exerted over an area.

**Pulmonary hypertension:** an increased blood pressure within the pulmonary circulation.

**Pulmonary oedema:** the escape of fluid into the air sacs and interstitial tissue of the lungs.

**Regulator:** a device for reducing air pressure.

**Repetitive dive:** any dive that is performed whose decompression profile is affected by retained inert gas of a previous dive. Usually in recreational diving, this means dives are done on the same day.

**Rhinorrhoea:** discharge from the nose.

**Safety stop:** a non-mandatory stop on ascent from a dive to allow additional off-gassing and reduce the risk of decompression illness.

**Sarcoidosis:** systemic granulomatous disease of unknown origin.

**Scoliosis:** a rotatory lateral curvature of the spine.

**Scuba:** self-contained underwater breathing apparatus.

**Second stage regulator:** the regulator that is held in the diver's mouth which reduces the pressure of the air at intermediate pressure from the first stage to the ambient pressure so the diver can breathe with ease.

**Sinuses:** air spaces within the skull.

**Spasticity:** increased tone or rigidity of a muscle.

**Spina bifida:** congenital defect in which part of the vertebral column is absent.

**Spondylosis:** abnormal immobility and fixation of a vertebral joint.

**Vasoconstriction:** narrowing of the lumen of blood vessels, especially of the arterioles.

**Vasodilation:** widening of the lumen of blood vessels, especially of the arterioles.

**Ventricle:** a cavity, especially in the heart or brain.

**Vertigo:** the illusion of revolving movement.

**Water pressure:** the force per unit area exerted by the weight of water.

**Wetsuit:** a close-fitting suit, usually made of neoprene, which keeps the diver warm by insulating the diver and trapping a layer of water between the diver and the suit.

**Xiphoid process:** small triangular-shaped bone at the base of the sternum.

## ACRONYMS

| | |
|---|---|
| BSAC | British Sub Aqua Club |
| DAN | Divers Alert Network |
| DMAC | Diving Medical Advisory Council |
| ECHM | European Committee for Hyperbaric Medicine |
| EUBS | European Underwater & Baromedical Society |
| PADI | Professional Association of Diving |
| RSTC | Instructors Recreational Scuba Training Council |
| SPUMS | South Pacific Underwater Medical Society |
| SSA | Sub-Aqua Association |
| SSI | Scuba Schools International |
| TDI | Technical Diving International |
| UKSDMC | UK Sport Diving Medical Council |
| UHMS | Underwater Hyperbaric Medical Society |

# INDEX

## C



## D

# E



# F



# G

## Q



## R



## S

## T



## U



## V

## W